TRUCKING YOGA

SIMPLE FITNESS
FOR THE
LONG HAUL

TRUCKING YOGA

SIMPLE FITNESS
FOR THE
LONG HAUL

HOPE ZVARA
E-RYT500, CPT
FOUNDER, MOTHER TRUCKER YOGA

ILLUSTRATIONS BY STEVE WORTHINGTON

Disclaimer: You should consult your physician or other healthcare professional before starting this or any other fitness program to determine if it is right for your needs. This is particularly true if you have a history or family history of high blood pressure or heart disease, or if you have ever experienced chest pain when exercising or have had chest pain in the past month when not engaged in physical activity, smoke, have high cholesterol, are obese, or have a bone or joint problem that could be made worse by a change in physical activity. Do not start this fitness program if your physician or healthcare provider advises against it. If you experience faintness, dizziness, pain, or shortness of breath at any time while exercising, you should stop immediately.

This book offers health and fitness information and is designed for educational purposes only. You should not rely on this information as a substitute for, nor does it replace, professional medical advice, diagnosis, or treatment. If you have any concerns or questions about your health, you should always consult with a physician or other healthcare professional. Do not disregard, avoid, or delay obtaining medical or health-related advice from your healthcare professional because of something you may have read here. The use of any information provided is solely at your own risk.

Developments in medical research may impact the health, fitness, and nutritional advice that appears here. No assurance can be given that the advice contained in this book will always include the most recent findings or developments with respect to the particular material.

If you are in the United States and think you are having a medical or health emergency, call 911 immediately.

ISBNs
Paperback edition: 978-1-947635-47-0
Ebook edition: 978-1-947635-48-7

CONTENTS

Introduction   1

Part I: Pride and Polish   5

1. The Convenience Trap   7
2. Health on Your Own Terms   18
3. A Strong Foundation: Your Posture and Core   31
4. 4 Essential Moves: Bend, Reach, Rotate, and Squat   45

Part II: In-Cab Fitness: Get Fit While You Sit   72

5. You in the Driver's Seat   74
6. Sleeper, Not Just for Sleeping   86
7. Outside Your Rig   108

Never Lose Hope   133

Resources   134

Acknowledgments   135

About the Author   136

Contact Hope   138

"A man too busy to take care of his health is like a mechanic too busy to take care of his tools."
—*Spanish Proverb*

INTRODUCTION

I am not a truck driver. I didn't grow up around trucking, and my husband does not drive an 18-wheeler. I am the daughter of a sewer pipe layer—you know, the man sixty feet down in the hole wading in raw sewage fixing our country's underground piping system so we can take showers, flush toilets, and live civilized lives the way we do. Yeah, that's me.

Growing up, all I saw was hard work. My father did not have a glamorous job, but he was good at it. And eventually, the physical demands of his career, coupled with not taking the best care of himself, led him to retire early with the label of disability on his shoulders. For years I wondered why he wouldn't go back to physical therapy or exercise or get a gym membership. Something. But after botched surgeries, all he ever knew was ripped out from under him. When he was no longer able to live up to the "I can get 'er done" lifestyle, I understood why.

I found yoga out of my own struggles with addiction, and yoga became my constant light. Yoga reminded me that there was hope, and through understanding how to breathe and live in this thing we call a body, I was able to fully recover and went from yoga student to yoga teacher.

As a yoga teacher I watched so many bodies move that I have discovered and learned about the body and how we move, not how to exercise, but how we move, breathe, and feel. I learned how everything we do on the yoga mat is a mirror for our everyday lives. Slowly over the years, my approach to yoga and fitness changed from memorizing poses to having a better understanding of people, and I saw the gaps—the gaps between our everyday lives and coming to yoga (or the gym).

We didn't need more yoga; we needed more yoga in our everyday lives. More daily movement, more daily breathing, more time spent feeling rather than stuffing everything down, and topping it with a smile. I wanted to change this approach to health, fitness, and wellness but didn't feel the yoga community was where I was meant to do that.

One November evening in 2017 changed everything.

My husband invited me to come to a local business mixer just outside my small hometown of Hartford, Wisconsin, and while we were at this mixer, a man walked up to my cocktail table and struck up a conversation. I had never met him; I knew 99 percent of the people in that room, but not him. We started talking, and I tried to pitch him corporate wellness for his employees in the office.

With a dead stare, he looked at me and said, "Do you have anything for truck drivers, like in the cab of their truck?"

I threw my hands in the air and said, "Mother Trucker Yoga!"

My now former business partner immediately stuck out his hand and said, "I love it, want to go into business together?"

I had just met this man, and now I was shaking his hand. That night two perfect strangers became business partners.

He was in trucking, and I was in yoga, and over the next four months, we built a company from scratch. During that time, something unique happened. I found my place. I may not have grown up around a semi-truck, but I understand the body, I know hardship, I know what it takes to change your life when you feel like there is no hope. If you want someone to teach you about trucking, ask a truck driver; if you want someone to teach you about improving your life and the body you live in within the trucking industry, that's where I come in.

I have made it my mission to impact the lives of those in the trucking industry. I show them through small, simple changes with activities they can do in five minutes or less how they can move the needle in their health and wellness.

As for my father, he spent years of his life living in pain and barely interacting with his surroundings. In the last year, however, something switched for him. He may not be in the best of health, and there are many things broken about him that are unfixable. But this man has changed his life for the better. Walking miles a day, drinking water, eating better, moving more—today he is a part of my life in a way he hasn't been in twenty-five years.

He's a changed person. Not because of a gym or a yoga mat, but because he built a toolbox of everyday life tools and uses them every day.

I want that for you too.

This book will help you understand how to take back the body you live in step by step. Life is meant to be enjoyed, so movement and exercise should not be seen as punishment, it should be seen as a joyful expression of living. Inside this book I want to create a simple understanding of how to move, when to move, and where to move for you as a truck driver. I want to simplify things. I want to pull you out of the weeds of confusion and help you to see that you can actively live life as a truck driver and be healthy as you do it.

Why Mother Trucker Yoga?

Mother Trucker Yoga may just be a fun name I came up with on a whim during a conversation with a stranger. But Mother Trucker Yoga is also an accumulation of everything I have learned and everything I believe, while being 100% me, and it just so happens my passion is with truck drivers. It's twenty years of learning, growing, and decoding everything that was confusing to me about the yoga and fitness world.

For years I'd dive into new aspects of fitness and health, but there was always a part of me that just didn't feel it was where I belonged. A part of me knew that that world wasn't where I belonged. I never fell in love with the hype of fancy poses or fed into the fancy yoga style fads, and although yoga helped me on many levels, that help had nothing to do with being a perfect yogi and everything to do with figuring out who I am and learning to take better care of my body.

I've read dozens of books, taken dozens of trainings and certifications, and have worked with thousands of real live humans, and after all of that I was still left wondering why so many people don't move more. I discovered that many of us have put movement into a box. We live our lives and only during this very specific time of the day or week will we move more. You've got it all wrong. Our lives are meant to be full of movement, and I am determined to show you how.

Mother Trucker Yoga may have emerged from a random conversation that turned into a new business adventure, but really I believe it's where I belong. I define Mother Trucker Yoga as my practical understanding of how the body moves, a philosophy that is combined with my own life struggles and the pieces of yoga that helped me to overcome them, mixed with the rawness of the trucking world. When I say I get to be me with Mother Trucker Yoga, I mean it. And when you come and join the movement over at Mother Trucker Yoga, what you get is an understanding and a toolbox to live a life worth moving for.

PART I:

PRIDE AND POLISH

Truckers love their rigs. We have all seen that blinged-out semi driving down the interstate, the rigs with the decorative lights, the colors, and accessories, like chrome or extra exhaust pipes. Some drivers spend thousands of dollars to deck out their rig to make it stand out.

If you have been to a truck show, there is usually a section called Pride and Polish, the Miss America of the trucking industry. Judges rate drivers' trucks in categories like most chrome, most lights, interior, exterior, tires/wheels, driver presentation, engine, and more. Drivers put a lot of time, energy, and effort into preparing their trucks for everyone to see. They travel for miles to show off their pride and joy at shows. When you roam around and view these delicacies at these events, you will understand why drivers put so much into cleaning, waxing, and polishing every inch of their big rig for spectators to ogle at these artworks on wheels.

Many drivers put all their attention into their rig, but they ignore their own health, and drivers don't have it easy. They are twice as likely as the average American to smoke, have obesity or diabetes, and have an increased risk of dying from health difficulties. Less than 6 percent of drivers grade their health as excellent, very good, or even good. That's terrible!

The problem is this: the trucking community needs truck drivers to survive. Now some will say autonomous trucks will soon dominate the industry, but you and I both know driverless trucks will never completely take over and definitely not anytime soon. The current challenge is for drivers to see their health as valuable. They must make a shift to giving their own health the same time, energy, and effort as they put into maintaining their truck.

What if you took just a few minutes a day to polish yourself up when it comes to your health and well-being? That truck wasn't built in a day, and getting it ready to enter it into a Pride and Polish trucking show also didn't happen overnight. Your health is no different.

Does this task seem overwhelming? How do we eat an elephant? One bite at a time. I want to invite you to a new way of looking at your health and fitness, one bite at a time. So the next time a truck show comes along, you will be standing next to your truck not to just take pride in your ride, but in the person who drives it, too.

Warning! What you are about to read may not be as glamorous as other lifestyle programs. And will most likely cause you to see being healthy as simple. So if you want something more exciting, something with complex equipment or high-intensity workouts or strict meal plans, something shinier, stop reading this book right now and give this book to another driver who you feel may need it.

1. THE CONVENIENCE TRAP

Once we humans roamed the hills hunting and gathering our own food and then taking the time to prepare, cook, and eat it in that same environment. Today, hunting and gathering has been replaced with faster and more convenient methods. As convenient as it may seem, our technology-based culture has outsourced nearly all our daily movement patterns more than ever before. Modern culture has fallen to its most significant disease—not cancer, diabetes, or mental health challenges—the disease of outsourced movement.

And it is the most significant disease we can contract. Lack of movement infiltrates every aspect of our lives, and when we try to fight it, we are tagged as being from the stone age or told to work harder, not smarter. Sure, farming advancements, industrial improvements, and even all of our social upgrades have made some tasks better, but at what cost?

I'm talking about modern conveniences. With obesity at an all-time high in our country, it isn't just food that's to blame. It's the introduction of gadgets, gizmos, and technology. Remember when you had to get up to change the channel on the TV or when you wanted to bake a cake and you had to mix the batter by hand? Or when getting outside and walking around was not seen as a waste of time? The problems caused by lack of movement are an accumulation of the little things over time. The little things we do for our health and well-being and an accumulation of the actions we are no longer doing for our health and well-being.

You can move more. You just choose not to, and when you have the option to walk, carry, skip, squat, reach, or bend, you are choosing not to. As a society, we are so focused at measuring the cells in our body for internal disease that we are missing the disease right under our noses.

There are two sides to every coin. You become whatever you surround yourself with. It's contagious. So if you are pursuing a lifestyle you no longer want or habits you know aren't good for you, I'm glad you picked up this book. Because everything in here is as contagious and simple to contract as catching a cold.

Is Good Health Even Possible over the Road?

Do truck drivers want to improve their health? Yes, but for most, a healthy driver is not the first concern that comes to mind when scheduling a load or figuring out how certain goods will make it from California to New York. If you are sick or your truck isn't running, there is no paycheck. Money is motivation inside trucking, as companies offer sign-on bonuses.

At the same time, companies outside trucking draw in new workers with extensive wellness plans and excellent healthcare options besides those potential bonuses. I've worked in schools and with large corporations providing wellness seminars, classes, and services. There is a clear incentive from the company for employees to keep healthy and fit. But for truck drivers, that incentive is rare.

Because truck stops are shifting away from dine-in food to fast-food, some drivers no longer have healthier food options. At a mini-

The Results Are In:
Sitting Is Bad for Your Health

The long-term effects of sitting four or more hours per day (as reported by GetAmericaStanding.org) would lead to these situations:

- Enzymes responsible for burning harmful blood fats to shut down

- Reduced calorie burning (lower metabolic rate)

- Disrupted blood sugar levels

- Increased insulin and blood pressure levels

- Leg muscles switching off

No matter your level of physical activity, the result of sitting leads to increased risks for these health conditions:

- Heart disease
- Diabetes
- Obesity
- Cancer
- Backache
- Dementia
- Depression
- Muscle degeneration

mum, the shift has made it a bit more difficult to grab a healthy bite when stopping at certain truck stops. And with personal safety an increasing issue, it's not always optimal to get out and exercise at some of those truck stops.

For most of America, going to the gym and going on a diet is what we equate to living a fit and healthy lifestyle. But for drivers, those two activities have a few more speed bumps along the way than for most of America. Why? Grabbing a healthy bite to eat isn't as easy as a quick run to the grocery store on the way home from work, or meal prepping for the entire week, because not every truck has a refrigerator in it. And heading to their favorite gym or yoga studio after work isn't possible for most drivers who often sleep in a different town each night.

Fitness Means Going to the Gym (No, Not Really)

I met Mark several years ago through a friend. He drove a day cab around town and appeared to take good care of himself. He was a healthy weight, did not seem to struggle when hopping in and out of his truck, and in our first conversation, he shared with me that he lifted weights and worked out every day. My initial thought was, "Wow, this guy's got game."

But later I learned something critical about his current health. His daily work life involved a lot of sitting, immobile, with short bursts of activity when loading and unloading. After work, he was diligent with weightlifting, toning, and cardio, but did very little to nothing for increasing mobility and flexibility. He was stiff, could hardly bend forward, and his shoulders had a minimal range of motion.

I asked Mark a fundamental question you might ask yourself: "How healthy do you feel?"

His response (and maybe yours), "Great, but—"

That is always my first clue that things are not as they seem. Mark looked fit and healthy, but his body was telling him otherwise. Sure, he could lift heavy luggage and cargo, but he couldn't function in his everyday life with ease. He couldn't do the activities he needed and wanted during the day without discomfort. Is that healthy? Is that fit? I believe the answer is no.

I was just like Mark, believing that achievement on the yoga mat equaled health. There came a point in my yoga practice and career where I realized several of the yoga poses I was teaching had nothing to do with keeping my body healthy and fit.

- Why am I teaching students to stand on their heads when most can't even stand on one foot, let alone two?
- What good is mastering a fancy twist if you still can barely reach back to grab your seat belt without making a squeamish face?

I wanted to better understand how we move and how we don't move. I wanted to see my students move closer toward wellness in ways that improved their daily lives, not just their yoga practice. And to do that, I needed to change my approach to fitness, yoga, and life.

Now this thinking might go against everything society has taught you about health and fitness. But hear me out. As we age, big muscles, speedy run times and mastering fancy moves will not win the race of independence and optimal health as we age. In today's world, whether you're a truck driver, a schoolteacher, or an accountant, we sit too much. And when we are not sitting, the movement patterns we take on to improve our health and well-being are often not efficiently balancing out what our body needs and our environment lacks.

As a culture, we do not need more exercise to solve our health crisis. Doing 30 minutes of exercise a day is a drop in the bucket when there are 1,440 minutes in a day. That's a whopping 2.08 percent of the day you spend in "exercising." Stop telling yourself that you already worked out, so you are all set for the day. That is the wrong mentality to have toward your body's physical and mental health.

It might surprise you to find that, even as a truck driver, within your everyday routine, you have ample opportunities to get moving throughout your day. In math sometimes you need a new formula to find the answer. Little movements all day long often equal more movement than going to the gym.

Suppose you can run for miles but cannot even bend down to put on your shoe. That's a problem. Maybe you can do 100 push-ups but are as stiff as a board and you can barely get your arms up over your head. That's not being fit and healthy. Fitness does not equal exercise.

Fitness is fitting movement into your everyday life. Fitness means fitting motion into your life with energy and happiness, as well as doing the activities you need to do and want to do, and seeing your daily life as an opportunity to celebrate how your body moves. Fitness is a unit of measurement that we can use to gauge our body's health.

Before we go any further, I need to say something. I am not against exercise. I think pumping iron in a gym and running a few miles on a treadmill and getting to a yoga class is a super-duper essential and significant addition to living a healthy life. For some, fitness should be about reclaiming the body they are currently living in.

We Defer Maintenance

My mom's van recently broke down on the side of the road. The electrical went haywire, and the check-engine light and every other light was flashing. The engine was making a funny noise, and the smell of something burning was coming from under the hood. It was no longer functioning optimally.

My dad had the van towed to our back shop, and after a day of letting the vehicle sit, my dad turned the key, and to our surprise, the van was running. He drove it up and down the street a few times, and it seemed as if nothing had ever happened.

I share this story because many of us treat our bodies the same way. With an ache or a pain, our bodies tell us something is not right. Then the symptom goes away, and suddenly, we have forgotten that something happened. Because things appear to be okay, we go on with our lives. There was, without a doubt, something wrong with that van. The smell of something burning was not good. That was a warning sign from the van fairy that my mom needed to stop and look closer.

But who wants to spend the time, the energy, or the money to look into a problem if it appears to be okay right now?

That van was not functioning the way it was designed it to run. Are you? Are you functioning safely? Are you functioning efficiently? Are you moving the way you are designed? Do you have a dashboard light flashing?

A big rig has eighteen wheels running fast and hard and carries a load maxed out at 80,000 pounds. If one of those gigantic tires blows, each wheel is designed to pick up the slack—in a built-in (temporary) backup plan. Truckers prepare for any environment by adding safety devices like chains to gain better traction, grip, and control in unpredictable environments or by organizing their load in the trailer to ensure adequate weight distribution for a safe haul.

Every driver I have ever met in the trucking community is running fast and hard. For some drivers, the maxed-out load is not the one on eighteen wheels; it's the one in the driver's seat.

Truckers are frequently up against the elements on the open road— elements such as healthy food availability, limited space, limited time, and the constant pressure of uncertainties that come with truck driving, such as traffic, the security of loads, Mother Nature, and what riding over a scale at a weigh station might do to their time line.

All too often, we wait to take care of our bodies. We wait until the last minute to mend something that we know has been breaking for years— our knees, backs, guts, feet, and even our minds. We think we can run on empty for a few more days until we get where we are going. We promise ourselves that we're going to take care of that dashboard light. But we immediately busy ourselves with other priorities.

We are living, then, a life of temporary fixes, but can we afford another tire to blow? You may be thinking that the only way to improve your fitness is to change careers or move or wait until your kids are older or any number of excuses. Know this: If you cannot change your environment,

For your own body's tune-up, are you are telling yourself you'll do it tomorrow? Or once you get a new job? Or when your kids are older? Or once the truck stops, or when you have more space to work out? Or when debts are paid off? Or when your employer allows you to take your health more seriously? Or my ultimate favorite: when you have more time?

All the excuses I hear have one thing in common (yes, those are all excuses). All those responses deal with something outside yourself. When those words come out of your mouth, you, my friend, are saying that your health, your well-being, and your tune-up are someone else's responsibility. And when you hand that responsibility to someone else, you give your power away; you give someone else priority over your life.

I know about this because I did this for years. I struggled for my life as I limped my way into recovery from a life-strangling addiction and a slew of mental health issues. I wondered why I couldn't get well. And attached to every one of those thoughts and statements was a reason someone else or something else was keeping me there. The moment you take responsibility for your life, you own it. When you say no more, enough is enough, mean it. Things can finally change.

When you assign blame to another, you lose some power and momentum to change those things yourself. A part of your brain decides that it is not your responsibility. You give up before you even try. You may not like your current situation, but you cannot change something you are not first aware of.

Much like you as a responsible driver should inspect the truck, trailer, lines, clamps, nuts, mounting brackets, locking jaws, locking pins, and bolts, the same should go for your body. You must inspect your own body's health regularly before going out on the road, not just the health of your truck.

please know you can change how you live and move in your environment today. It is about the small, simple changes that will lead you down the road to a healthier, happier, more fit you.

I Already Have Health Problems

Now I know what you are thinking: "But, Hope, I had a knee replacement, or I have a herniated disk, or I have high blood pressure, or a bad back." I want to validate that. Except before this pain, discomfort, or problem, did your check-engine light go on? Did you hear a clunking noise and do nothing? Did your system go haywire, and then seem fine, so you went on driving? Are you broken down on the side of your life, and you keep trying to limp along?

Is what you are doing now sustainable? Is the way you move about your day, the exercise routine you are currently following, sustainable for the long haul?

Considering the current track you are on, when you reach the age of eighty will you be able to live and function optimally and independently throughout the day? If you want to reach up and grab that cup out of the high cabinet, are you currently able to do it? Can you efficiently do it now? If you're going to squat down and pick up your shoe or that bag on the floor, are you able to do so now? If you want to twist and rotate to do simple things like buckle up or pull something from behind, are you doing it now? Can you quickly do it now? If you want to keep your independence and put on your shoes, pants, and socks, are you doing it now? Can you quickly do it now?

If you want to end up in a wheelchair when you are elderly, keep sitting. You can combat all that sitting with small, simple inserts of movement throughout your day. Yes, even while driving. You can do exercises while sitting in your environment, and those exercises will make a difference now and later.

Think of someone you know who is eighty or ninety years old. What do you know about them? How do they move? How do they not move? What do they do during the day? What don't they do during the day? What is a day in the life of Aunt Helen or Uncle Joe like?

It doesn't have to be sedentary and debilitating. This shift doesn't mean a radical change in career or an impossible commitment to crazy exercises. It means you decide you want to listen in and are ready to get your van running again so you can go on living. Are you in?

Your Body's Aches and Pains Self-Care Check-In

Pull out that piece of paper now, and do me a favor, write how you feel. What's going wrong? What's going right? What exactly is your body telling you right now? Write down everything. Do not judge the words, experiences, and feelings that come out onto the paper.

When assessing your body, you want to ask yourself: Am I moving closer to wellness or closer to pain? Are my actions responding to my body's feelings, calls, and requests? Take a few minutes and check in with your body and notice how you feel.

❑ Are your feet sore? Stiff? Tender? Like they are on pins and needles?

❑ Are your ankles stiff?

❑ Are your knees weak? Stiff? Unwilling to do what you ask? In pain? Unstable? Unreliable? Feeling a pinch when you sit, walk, or move?

❑ Are your legs weak? Stiff? Sore? Tingling? Achy? Do you feel pinching? In pain?

❑ Do your hips ache? Feel stiff? Sore? Weak? Lack full range of motion? Do they creak? Pop or click?

❑ Does your tailbone hurt? Throb? Ache?

❑ Does your back feel stiff? Sore? Achy? Throb? Are there shooting sensations? Is it hard to stand up straight? Twist? Or bend?

❑ Do your shoulders hurt? Are they sore? Stiff? Immobile? Click, pop, or creak? Is there numbness or tingling?

❑ Does your neck ache? Feel stiff? Sore? Lack range of motion? Pinch? Throb?

- [ ] Are your arms weak? Tingling? Sore? Throbbing? Stiff?

- [ ] Are your hands weak? Losing grip strength? Tingling? Sore? Stiff? Tender?

- [ ] Does your jaw clench? Grind? Lock?

Answering yes to any of the questions might mean it's time for a wellness pit stop—a head-to-toe tune-up. And the good news, you can start this tune-up today. Are you willing and ready? You only get one body, and replacement parts are never as good as the originals.

Now that you have taken an inventory of your body's current state and documented it on paper, read it back out loud. You need to hear your voice say these observations. And do not assign blame. Do not point any fingers at anyone. Once you take ownership, from there you can tune up this fantastic vehicle called the human body.

Changing Lanes for Trucker Health

What if drivers and trucking companies showed the same concern for their health as they do for their rigs and the loads they carry? What if every trucker in America (all 3.5 million of you) preserved their bodies the same way as they do their rigs? What if the 1.2 million trucking companies in the U.S. saw drivers' good health as necessary as the trucks they ride in?

Maintaining a healthy lifestyle as a truck driver is not the norm; many drivers live in their truck for a week to six weeks to six months at a time. And since I have been working with drivers, it has become clear it's not about giving them meals to eat or offering them gym time. Healthy living has to start at the beginning by laying out how each driver can set a healthy base for living—no matter where they are.

I've seen the transformations. When drivers invest the same time, energy, and effort into their health as they do their truck's health and visual appeal, they also become more capable behind the wheel. But there is a portion of the trucking community that identifies as being rough and tough cowboys. When I suggest they should consider health, fitness, or yoga, they laugh.

When I first started Mother Trucker Yoga and went to my first truck show, I did not know what to expect. Overall, the response was positive; drivers, family members of drivers, and other trucking company owners thanked me for what I am doing. But mixed in were the tried-and-true die-hard cowboys. The way they moved screamed that they needed a little yoga in their lives, but they would be damned if they would ever be caught dead doing yoga. They were set on avoiding being labeled with the misperception that yoga is about tight pants and crazy unnatural positions.

I believe we can change this stigma. Truck drivers and trucking companies can make a shift. The first step is to think that health—at least better health—is definitely possible over the road. We need to change lanes and try things differently. And to do that, we must rethink the limitations of our environments, our current circumstances, and our ingrained habits.

Change begins with something as simple as reading this book. Drivers and their counterparts must start focusing on the current issues facing the trucking community's health. So if the industry pivots toward a more health-conscious driver, and if everyone takes even just one step toward driver health, our truckers—the ones hauling our goods, our food, and our products—can change lanes regarding their health with less traffic along the way.

My goal is to show you how you can add all of that into your day and how you can tune up your life to tune up your body and your health. This book shows you where, why, and how to insert health, fitness, and wellness into your lifestyle, even as a truck driver.

2. HEALTH ON YOUR OWN TERMS

If you want to tune up your health, you first have to understand what health is. Most people measure health based on how they look, how they look on paper, or how they look compared to the rest of their family. You may hear words like "she looks healthy, because she is thin," or "his health is not great, because he has arthritis," or "he won't get better, because his father died young."

My point is none of these observations are worth holding onto or have anything to do with you. You should measure health based on how you feel.

Have you ever asked a blind person what health looks like to them? The CUT media and news channel did a video asking blind people what they think beauty is. In the video, they all said they saw beauty by the use of other senses and that it's not the vision (what's seen), it's the expression of their hearts, their whole experience. The base of everything they see comes from what they feel, while sighted people often base everything they see on sight alone.

Move as You Are Designed to Move

Our bodies are complex. We have many moving parts, and the majority of what moves and operates our bodies is beneath the surface. This tells us that what we see is not always the whole story. And over the past twenty years, I have come to understand that downplaying the body's remarkable systems and deeply interconnected parts is not something I want to do. But I do want to simplify it.

My first anatomy class in my first-ever yoga teacher training felt like it was conducted in French, and the only word I know in French is French toast. But there I was teaching yoga. It wasn't until several years later that I took it upon myself to learn people, not poses, so I could learn about how the body moves, and why, not just fancy yoga poses. And to save you time, energy, and confusion, here are three key points I want you to know after reading this book:

1. Your body is meant to move (research has proven this).

We are not designed to sit around. My husband always uses the philosophy of work smarter not harder. Use modern advancements to save your body from hardship and injury, but there is a line where convenience begins to rob us of the very gift our body gives us—movement.

Are you letting various pockets of time slip by where you could get up and get moving? Maybe you are saying it's because you don't have a sit-stand desk. So make one. Or maybe you are stuck in the driver's seat. Well you can move there, too. You can live, you can breathe, you can move inside your life right now. Stop waiting for some class or perfect opportunity.

When you move more, you breathe more, and that life force in your body is a major indicator of being alive. Moving about in your everyday life jump-starts your heart and every major system and organ in your body.

Not moving = Not breathing = Slowly dying
Moving = Breathing = Living

2. When you move, you also lubricate your joints and stretch your tissues.

The effects of long-term sitting on our tissues are like glue, hardened plastic, clumpy glue. The longer you go without moving, the more the glue sticks together. The layers and layers and layers of tissues (fascia, muscle, ligaments, tendons) all begin to clump together and cause stiffness, pain, immobility, and injury. And you didn't even do anything to create that problem.

That same immobility stops the natural lubricating effect that happens in your joints when you move. Those are the same joints that want to take you up the stairs and use to reach up over your head or bend down to put on a sock.

**Not moving = No joint lubrication and plastic-like tissues =
Increased injury
Moving = Joints lubricated and elastic-like tissues = Less injury**

3. When you move, you feel better.

When you move, you boost the feel-good chemicals and hormones in your brain that make you happy. I can't help but think about the mental health crisis in this country and how moving more could be the prescription we all need more of.

Do this: Get outside, go for a walk. Do ten squats every time you go to the bathroom. Roll your ankles while idling in traffic. Swing your arms like you are swimming until you can feel your heart thumping. For gosh sakes, smile, your face has muscles, too. If you want to feel better, nothing will do what movement can do for you. Stop thinking movement only comes in the package called exercise or from the gym or the yoga mat. Fit happens there, too. But it happens in your everyday life first.

**Not moving = Increased anxiety, depression, unhappiness
Moving = Increased happiness and living your life**

Your Healthy Body Check-In

Now close your eyes, take a deep breath, and take notice of what picture your mind paints. Would you be out playing in the backyard with your kids? Are you moving smoothly in and out of your truck? Would you be training for a 5k? Maybe you are a few pounds lighter. Would your skin look firm, glowing, and hydrated? Are you standing up tall, ready for what the day throws at you? Would your eyes look bright? Is there a smile on your face?

What does healthy feel like? I want to encourage you not to base what is healthy in your body solely on what is in the mirror. Close your eyes and use your other senses. Let's check in.

❑ When I wake up, I feel refreshed and fully rested.

❑ I can get in and out of my truck with ease.

❑ My clothes fit comfortably.

❑ My shoulders are down away from my ears.

❑ I have the energy to do what I need and what I love.

❑ I smile more than I frown.

❑ My muscles feel firm and willingly carry me throughout the day.

❑ My middle feels slender and void of restriction.

❑ My body moves freely.

❑ My mind is clear and alert.

❑ I stand tall.

❑ I can easily take a deep breath.

❑ My back feels strong and willing to take on the day.

If you feel that you need to lose weight for the sake of losing weight, what is it about the weight loss that you think will give you what you need or want in your health? Is it losing weight, or is it the freedom weight loss would give to your life? The ability to move with ease? No longer be out of breath? To be able to get down on the ground and play with your kids or grandkids? Or have more confidence when you go out in public?

If you desire to be more flexible, what is it about the flexibility you feel you need to be healthier? What will the increased flexibility offer you? Less fear of falling? More agility? The ability to move quickly and with ease? Or how about knowing that you can still put your pants, shoes, and socks on all by yourself for years to come?

Use the check-in here as mile markers, checkpoints along the way to help you assess your self-improvement goals and why you want those abilities. You may come to find that *healthy* is closer than you think.

Roadside Assistance

You can't fix a problem with your vehicle if you don't know what the problem is. Part of going to school to get your CDL (Commercial Driver's License) and driving with a trainer is to learn what to look for if your truck stops working properly. To learn the ins and outs of driving, loading, and unloading. And temporarily fix the issue or resolve it.

But none of this is possible if you don't know what you are looking for if you break down. And practice makes perfect, so the more you do what you were taught, the more those actions become automatic, and you will be catching problems long before they happen.

As a culture we often want to fix a problem without ever figuring out the actual problem by treating the symptoms. I believe you first need to stop, take a hot minute, step back, and figure out what the problem is. If you have a headache, for example, you take aspirin to get rid of the headache, but what if you first stop and think why you have that headache? Dehydration or too much screen time, hormonal imbalance, change in altitude, change in pressure? There are dozens of reasons why a headache occurs.

If you feel unhealthy, unfit, or unhappy, you need to upgrade your lifestyle: how you breathe, move, and go about your day. And my goal for you is not to drive you crazy in trying to figure it all out, but rather to create a new step in your response system, in how you assess the problem and request assistance in the future.

Your Body Is Like a Truck

The human body is fantastic. We are capable of so much. Have you ever stood in awe and amazement and watched a small baby learn to crawl, push up to standing, walk, or run? How do they know? As a mom of three, I have never stood at the other end of a room and called out to my child to activate their core or contract their glutes when my child was attempting to crawl or take that first step.

You were once that small child, using your entire body to pull up to standing and take that first step; you just knew how. You never once thought to activate your glutes, core, or leg muscles to achieve your goal of stability and mobility. You never thought about turning on a body part to reach your goal when you were ready; you just did it.

But if you have ever stepped into the exercise and fitness world, one truth is apparent: you work parts not people. You have your legs day, your arms day, your biceps exercises, and your core exercises. This type of mentality leaves people assuming that you work only parts of your body separately and never use the whole body. That is like saying when your truck is running that it can separately choose when to use the pistons or the timing belt or the spark plugs at any given time.

I am no mechanic, but in order for the truck to run optimally, the entire truck needs to be working together. A truck is not a truck when the pieces are all separate. A truck is a truck when all the pieces are working together.

Human Body = Truck

Each part has a specific purpose. Alone it doesn't do much, but when you put all the parts together, something amazing happens. You have a fully operational truck.

Human Body Part	Truck Part	Function	Brief Exercise
Brain	Computer for the motor (ECM)	Control center	Learning, puzzling, talking, meditation
Lungs	Air filters	Air intake for motor to run	Deep breathing
Heart	Spark plugs (gas engine) and pistons	Power generation center	Brisk walking, jumping jacks
Stomach	Gas tank	Fueling center	Drinking water, eating healthy foods
Bones	Frame of vehicle	Foundation everything is mounted to	Stair climbing, lifting things, body-weight exercises
Joints, muscles, cartilage, ligaments, connective tissues	(Air) Suspension: shocks, springs and struts bushings, control arms, stabilizer arms	Absorbs impact and allows for flexibility, makes a smoother ride	Gentle stretching, walking, lifting, pushing, pulling, biking
Blood, veins and vessels	Drivetrain and transmission (automatic or manual)	To transfer power	Walking, inverting, legs up the wall pose

Human Body Part	Truck Part	Function	Brief Exercise
Water	Vehicle fluids: coolant, power steering fluid, DEF fluid, diesel, brake fluid, blinker fluid	Necessary for complete function and optimal performance of all aspects of life/truck	Fill a gallon jug of water, lift it and drink it
Feet	Tires and rims (wheels)	Traction and movement	Get your shoes off, roll out your feet, walk barefooted

We Are Not Parts, We Are People

You can't separate out body parts and think they are acting alone, it's impossible. One part may work harder than another during a specific move or exercise, but you are never flying solo on any given move or exercise.

Like your truck, all parts need to be kept lubricated and maintained in good working condition, and like your truck, you do not need more exercise to solve a health crisis. What you need is a better understanding of how to work efficiently and optimally as a whole. To be frank, we all need to get up off our behinds and get moving. And that movement needs to be an equal opportunity for your entire body and span the course of your day.

Are You Moving Closer to Wellness?

The first step in the process of assessment is redefining what health is, what being fit means, and what it can look like as a trucker. Health is you being an active part of a life worth living. When I think of being healthy or what it means to be fit, I think about what it takes to actively participate in my life. I'm not sitting on the sidelines watching. And it's equally as much about moving throughout the day and doing what needs to be done with ease so my daily life is not a struggle.

You may lift 500 pounds or run a marathon, but is your daily life and how you move through it done with ease, grace, and fluidity? I see health, fitness, and wellness (call it what you want) on a sliding scale, and every day I ask myself this one question: Am I moving closer to wellness or further away?

This question requests that you take inventory of the day and look at not just what you are doing, but how you are doing it.

Moving closer toward wellness means your knees don't hurt and your back isn't constantly stiff because you're sitting too much. And if that is the case, what are you doing about it?

For me, I am making healthier food choices, even when it's hard. It's me walking and talking on my phone because there isn't any good reason not to be. It's me choosing to drink a large cup of water in the morning even when I don't want to, along with not buying junk food. It's me getting up and playing with my kids or stopping to stretch my back before I lift something heavy even when everyone is waiting for me because I know my body will be better for it.

What are you doing every day to move toward wellness?

When you wipe all the other stuff away, your body, your mind, and the way you move and breathe happen without a struggle. No matter how pretty the glass vase is, if there is a crack in it, the health of the vase is compromised. No amount of paint, glue, or turning it so no one sees the crack is going to change the fact that the health of the vase has been reduced.

Think of us as a sponge. If you don't squeeze it out, eventually that sponge is going to get slimy and gross, it will start to fall apart and no longer be a useful sponge. It's easier to throw the sponge in the sink and deal with it later or even throw it away. But if you just take a few moments to clean it after each use, that sponge can last with proper care. Isn't it time you squeezed out your sponge? That's bridging the gap in your health and fitness, squeezing your sponge after every use.

To help make health more accessible to drivers, it's about identifying the pockets of time throughout the day to sneak in movement, fitness, and health. It's about figuring out what you can do every single day. Ask yourself about any activity or inactivity or choice you make each day:

- Is it good for my health?
- Is it better than the alternative?
- Is it the best thing I can do for my body?

You may not be able to have the best of everything every single day. But do not let that keep you from moving the needle closer to wellness. No one is perfect, and your health and fitness does not need to be perfect. No one says it has to be. But I know there is something you can do today that is better than what you have done up to this point.

Better is you eating fast-food and getting a burger without a bun, or asking the manager if they can make a salad and put a grilled piece of chicken on top even though it's not on the menu. Better is walking laps around your truck even though there is no fitness center nearby and you don't even own walking shoes.

And choosing something healthier to eat or do means you are thinking of your health. Is this good for me? The best options might not be available and there might not be anything better. But this in front of me, this is good today. Good is walking more, good is buying a bag of nuts and a piece of fruit instead of a Snickers. Good is moving your body when your back screams at you—your back needs that movement to feel good. Good is you no longer making excuses because you are a truck driver.

If you want health, you will find a way to be healthy. When you shift your thinking to see what good choices are out there and how simple it can be to integrate them, living a fit and healthy lifestyle doesn't feel so out of reach.

The Pocket Effect

Idella was one of my first clients when I stepped into the trucking world. Idella is a trucking matriarch and has been behind the wheel since she was eighteen. Now, in her late sixties, she isn't slowing down. But when I first met with her, she said she felt stiff, her joints hurt, and she felt that arthritis was to blame.

After a few weeks of working through my video library and a few group check-ins, her situation improved. After about six months of following my straightforward process of adding more movement into her day—a few simple movements, many of which she did in her truck even while driving—her pain went away. Her joints no longer hurt, and she could move around more easily. All of this because of a few minutes a day.

It's been over two years since we first worked together, and Idella still uses these techniques, she is still trucking, and the best part is that she has connected the dots between being healthy and fit and moving more in her everyday life.

Any small thing you do to improve your health, fitness, and well-being is a step in the right direction.

There was a time when I felt tremendous guilt and was killing myself to be fit and healthy. From the outside, I was what our culture tells us is healthy. But I was stressed, exhausted, and beating myself up when I didn't exercise for two or more hours a day. That wasn't healthy. That was the definition of insanity.

For years I continued to eat vegan when my body was craving more. Because I was a yogi, that's what I thought that I should do. I got to a point where I either was going to break or reframe my health. After years of learning and trying out different methods, I discovered that it's not about putting my health and fitness into a box where I check off the exercise box and now I'm good. But it is about increasing the total amount of movement I do throughout the entire day.

I stepped back and looked at what I was doing and what I was teaching and saw the gap. The gap in my life and the lives of many others had to do with what we were doing to be fit and healthy—our effort at checking that box was putting us in a box. And we were only pulling out that box for a few minutes a day. That's the gap. And I saw that to live healthy and fit, we needed to bridge that gap.

Instead of shoving a lot of movement into one small period within twenty-four hours, let's expand the movements throughout the hours we are awake. Break the idea of exercise into small movements and fit them into pockets of time throughout your day. We all have these pockets of time, truck driver or not, and we all can move more, yet we don't. We tell ourselves, "I'm going to work out later" and because of that, we keep sitting around. Or we feel that backache or look at our bodies and think we need to exercise. At that moment we could get up and do something, but we do nothing.

You could get up and walk around. Do a few squats, use your water bottle as a hand weight. Stretch. And the moment your body feels discomfort, don't just stop at thinking about it. Get up and do something about it. The reality is one to five minutes will make a world of difference. What if you found five one-minute to five-minute pockets of time throughout your day? That's five to twenty-five minutes more activity every day.

When others see a kitchen sink, I see something to squat down and hang on to stretch my back. When others see a truck step, I see a place to stretch and an instant cardio machine. When others see a parking lot, I see a walking track to get your steps in. When others see a gallon of water, I see a hand weight to lift and then drink up afterward.

Your Daily Get Fit Quick Check-In

Fitness doesn't have to be complicated, and this checklist helps you see where you can add more movement into your day. Are you choosing convenience over simple solutions? Let's check in.

- ❏ When you pull into a parking lot, instead of finding the closest spot, park as far away as you can so you can walk more.

- ❏ When you put on shoes, bend down and use your hands to get your shoe on.

- ❏ When you eat something, instead of stuffing yourself with a burger in one hand and fries in the other, eat more deliberately by using a fork, knife, and spoon and cut your food.

- ❏ When you have free time, get up and move around, walk and talk on the phone, choose an activity instead of sitting down.

- ❏ When your body hurts, move, stretch, breathe, and work to ease the pain instead of popping a pain reliever pill.

- ❏ When you're driving, move around, safely stretch, and stay mobile.

- ❏ When you have the choice of the drive-thru or a walk-in restaurant, get out of your vehicle and move.

For the next twenty-four hours, pay attention to what you do and, most importantly, how you do it. By assessing yourself with the checklist, you can begin to take an inventory of not just what you do daily, but how you do things daily. Can you do what you are doing differently? In a new, more active way? Walk and talk? Sit and still move around? Start to improve those actions and you will begin to see your life transform.

3. A STRONG FOUNDATION: YOUR POSTURE AND CORE

Your posture is your foundation. Like a house, if the foundation is faulty, crooked, or has cracks and weak points, the house will show it. Leaks and drywall cracks leak energy, which is nearly unseen to the naked eye, but very much there.

Your body is no different. As you go about your day, pay attention to how you sit in the driver's seat after a few hours of driving. Notice how you stand in line or at the pump. Pay close attention to how you walk and move your body. Do you have special ways of doing things?

See if you can incorporate the following 5-Point Safety Check into your day while you are sitting, standing, walking, and moving about and notice what comes naturally and what isn't as natural. Focus on one point at a time until the behaviors become automatic. Check your chin while driving every hour. Take notice of the direction of your feet while standing or walking and correct them until you don't even have to think about it anymore. If you are walking forward, your feet should be pointing forward. You don't need to do all of these things right away. Instead, do one until it's a new healthy habit. And before you know it, you'll pass your posture inspection with flying colors.

A big piece of your posture pie is your core. Now this area of the body is not one muscle, but rather layers of muscles, going underneath you, wrapping around you, and going deep enough to attach to your spine, ribs, hips, and pelvis. I want to share a few key points with you to help you use and activate your core in all that you do.

Core Caution

Fitness trainers use many phrases when directing exercisers to use their core muscles that can be confusing and misleading. And this happens because most people using the phrases are not quite sure themselves. As

Standing 5-Point Safety Check

How you move is based on your body's posture. Improve your daily posture, and how you move will most certainly improve. When you first begin to improve your standing posture, please note that your body may fatigue, feel sore, and even cramp because you use muscles and body parts that have been asleep for quite some time. To start, pick one of the Standing 5-Point Safety Check Points and work on that until it becomes automatic. Then add another. Before you know it, they will all be automatic, and you will be moving better every day.

1. Point your feet forward, spread your toes and anchor down into all four corners of your feet.

2. Rotate legs slightly out (external rotation) so the slits on the backside of the knees point back, this should make your glutes contract.

3. Tip your pelvis into neutral, where the top of your pelvis feels level and the front hip bones and pubis bone are parallel with the front wall.

4. Allow your chest to open and shoulder blades to relax down, without popping your lower front ribs forward.

5. Slide your chin slightly in and your head back to feel the neck lengthen over your shoulders.

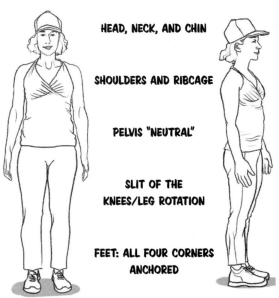

HEAD, NECK, AND CHIN

SHOULDERS AND RIBCAGE

PELVIS "NEUTRAL"

SLIT OF THE KNEES/LEG ROTATION

FEET: ALL FOUR CORNERS ANCHORED

Sitting 5-Point Safety Check

Sitting for any length of time can wreak havoc on the body. So use the Sitting 5-Point Safety Check to give your drivetime a tune-up. Depending on if you drive a manual or automatic, ideal body position may not always be possible. But use this Sitting 5-Point Safety Check to check in with your body and see what you can improve while driving to reduce pain and discomfort when you step out of the vehicle. Start with any one of the positions to keep your body in top-notch driving condition.

1. Place your pelvis level and sitting bones directly beneath the body (think untuck).

2. Gently arch the lower back away from the seat to bring back the natural curve of the lower back as you keep the belly gently toned.

3. Drop your shoulder blades down and back toward the spine.

4. Allow your chest to open and relax your arms down and the folds of the elbows to turn and face up.

5. Slide your chin slightly in and your head back to feel the neck lengthen over the shoulders.

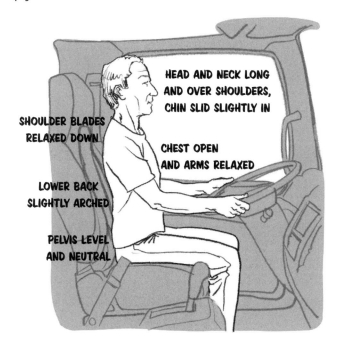

SHOULDER BLADES RELAXED DOWN

LOWER BACK SLIGHTLY ARCHED

PELVIS LEVEL AND NEUTRAL

HEAD AND NECK LONG AND OVER SHOULDERS, CHIN SLID SLIGHTLY IN

CHEST OPEN AND ARMS RELAXED

you read this book, I will use the phrases "activate your core" or "engage your core muscles." And when I say that, I mean the front, back, sides, top, and bottom of your middle. Your core is not one-dimensional. It is 360 degrees around and runs deep.

Your Core: Your core has multiple layers of muscle. And each of these muscles and the layers of muscle all work together. When specific muscles work harder than others, this can cause imbalance, pain, and even bodily injury. There is no single core muscle more critical than the next. Your core isn't just what you see on the outside. Always remember your core is made up of layers of muscle, not just one.

Your core includes:

- Your pelvic floor (bathroom muscles)—Your core's basement
- Your six-pack abs (rectus abdominis)—Your core's front wall
- Your sides (internal and external obliques)—Your core's side walls
- Your back muscles (the muscles running through and around your spine)—Your core's back walls

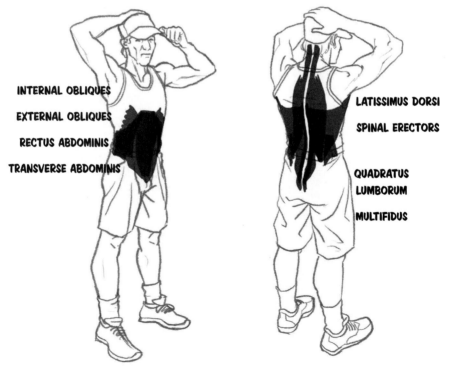

INTERNAL OBLIQUES

EXTERNAL OBLIQUES

RECTUS ABDOMINIS

TRANSVERSE ABDOMINIS

LATISSIMUS DORSI

SPINAL ERECTORS

QUADRATUS LUMBORUM

MULTIFIDUS

- Your transversus abdominis (which is a back muscle that wraps around you on the inside like a corset)—Your core's interior walls
- Your diaphragm (breathing muscle)—Your core's roof

I could write a whole manual on understanding your core (oh wait, I did), but for the sake of this pocket-style book I'm keeping the discussion of the core short and sweet.

Here's what you need to know about your core:

- Your core starts at your feet. Keep your feet healthy and mobile and your core will be too. It's all connected.
- Your pelvic floor matters. Practice long holds contracting your bottom (anal sphincter to urethra); there are muscles down there. Strengthening your pelvic floor is essential as you age (especially if you don't want to be peeing your pants). Think long holds rather than rapidly squeezing your pelvic floor muscles (known as Kegels or Kegel exercises) while you are driving, shopping, standing, or exercising.
- Cough and feel your entire core contract. That's what we want, not navel to spine.
- Your arms and legs are an extension of your core. Use them more, and you will use your core more. When you lift, carry, and reach, think about where the power is coming from.
- Improve your posture. Put your body back where it belongs, and your core muscles will automatically turn on as needed.
- Get your shoes off. The health of your feet is connected to the health of your physical body, and that includes the core. Stimulate your feet, stimulate your core.
- If you were a boxer and your opponent was about to punch you, what would you do? Not suck in, not push out, but you'd contract, you'd engage, you'd brace your core to take the blow. Be a boxer and engage your core.

- Do you want to experience your core engage? Put your hands on your waist and cough. Feel your core muscles contract. Now make a memory of that, and when someone asks you to contract your core, feel for that contraction.

Be the Bridge

Adult bodies have four curves. These curves are designed to create support, absorb impact and shock, create balance, distribute weight evenly, and help with a full range of motion. When we lose the spine curves, we also lose our body's ability to function optimally.

So do we have pain and discomfort because we are aging? Or do we have pain because of how we live in our bodies? Does our environment support the body we want to live in? How we do some things is how we do most things. And how we do most things is the accumulation of how we move about our day.

The truck, the driver's seat, the open road, and truck stop parking lots may be your environment now and in the foreseeable future, but that does not mean you can't change how you behave in them.

The Backbone of Good Posture

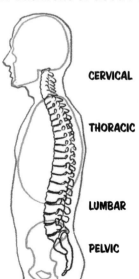

CERVICAL

THORACIC

LUMBAR

PELVIC

The spine is shaped in the form of an S curve for a reason: to create balance in your body and as a natural shock absorber. With the proper curvature, your body has the right balance of flexibility and support. With four curves each section holds its own importance: (1) Cervical–Neck, (2) Thoracic–Upper and Mid-Torso, (3) Lumbar–Lower Back, and (4) Pelvic, Sacrum–Hip Area.

Forty-two-pound Head

Lousy posture is like a dead weight you are carrying on your shoulders. That pain, discomfort, and tightness you feel in your upper back and shoulder blade area isn't your upper back's fault, and it isn't tightness. You've been carrying a bowling ball around in front of your body. And the more it rolls forward, the more pressure, pain, and strain it puts on the upper back muscles. Every inch your head falls forward increases the weight your neck and back muscles have to carry. Strain means those muscles are overstretched, most likely due to the weight of the forward head.

When your head is two inches forward from your shoulders you are putting roughly thirty-two pounds of pressure and strain on your neck, shoulders, and upper back. At three inches forward, you are looking at forty-two pounds of pressure and strain. That's a lot of extra weight to be carrying around like a bushel of apples attached and hanging down in front of you. Practice good posture and roll your head back where it belongs, on top of your shoulders.

YOUR HEAD GETS HEAVIER THE FURTHER FORWARD YOU GO

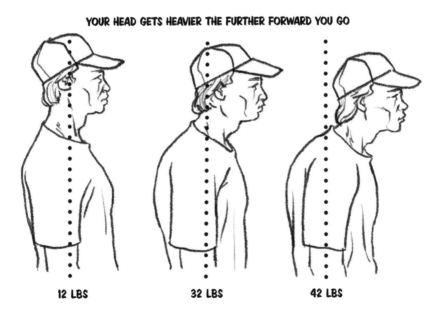

| 12 LBS | 32 LBS | 42 LBS |

Stand Up and Sit Up Tall

We adapt to our environment, so if your cab has a run-of-the-mill seat or a not-so-great seat, then your posture will reflect that. If you have a seat that doesn't help you maintain good posture, your body will remember it. And if you've been standing with poor posture, your body will remember that, too. Sitting and standing with good posture does not have to be complicated and is 100 precent broken down in the following pages.

WELLNESS PITSTOP CHECKLIST

Drive Your Way to Better Posture Check-In

All the movements and exercises you do throughout the day are performed based on your posture. When you improve your posture, your movements, and how you sit and go about your day in your environment, then how you live in that environment can change.

Take this Driver's Seat Check-In:

- ☐ Are you shifted onto one hip while sitting rather than keeping your hips level?

- ☐ Are you sitting on the top or center of your back pants pockets rather than sitting on the bottom edges?

- ☐ Is your lower back rounded back into the seat behind you?

- ☐ Is your upper back rounded and hunched away from the seat?

- ☐ Is your chest collapsed and chest muscles tight?

- ☐ Does your head hang forward from your shoulders?

- ☐ Does your upper back feel the strain after a short time driving?

- ☐ Does the impact from the truck leave you feeling stiff, sore, and beat up?

If you answered yes to any of the questions, it may be time for a posture tune-up.

When you begin to sit in better posture, this may also mean you have to tweak your environment. In this case, the truck seat. Utilizing something like a BackShield designed to support all the curves in your spine while driving may be an investment on the horizon if a new truck seat is not (review at www.BackShield.com).

Posturing

Your posture is essential. It's the foundation of how you move and don't move. Once you learn what type of posture you have, you can then work on self-correcting issues that cause problems. Do you identify with any of these types of postures?

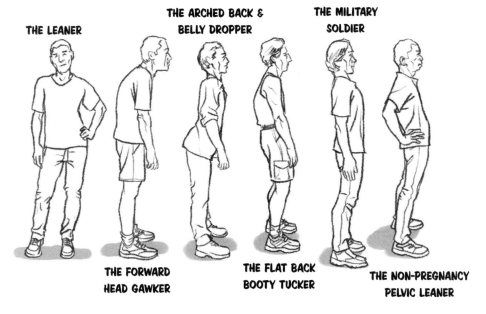

THE LEANER
THE ARCHED BACK & BELLY DROPPER
THE MILITARY SOLDIER
THE FORWARD HEAD GAWKER
THE FLAT BACK BOOTY TUCKER
THE NON-PREGNANCY PELVIC LEANER

The Leaner: Constantly leans into one hip. Possibly uses that hip to support objects and carry things. The sidekick stance creates a strain on ligaments and can shift and twist the pelvis while sliding the ribs and shoulders in the opposite direction, causing upper body strain and discomfort.

The Forward Head Gawker: Because of constant and continuous computer time, drive time, and hunching, the head now sits a few degrees to several inches forward of the shoulders. This position causes strain in the upper back and neck and rounded shoulders and shortens the pectoral muscles on the front of the body (also known as upper cross syndrome, kyphosis).

The Arched Back and Belly Dropper: A history of dramatic weight loss, pregnancy, or other injuries or issues may leave the body still behaving as it did previously. An imbalance of a weak core, glutes, and hamstrings, and a tight lower back can lead to numbness, tingling, and even sciatica.

The Flat Back Booty Tucker: With little spinal curvature, the body has little to no built-in shock absorbers to take on the impact of walking, running, jumping, even driving. This combination can cause a lack of stability in the pelvis and lumbar spine and even affect gait (how you walk).

The Military Soldier: The notion of "stand up straight" has left the neck and possibly other spine parts with little to no curvature. This curvature loss can cause an increase in spinal compression and degeneration. This loss in curvature can also cause balance and posture issues.

The Non-pregnancy Pelvic Leaner: The stance of choice involves a forward pelvic thrust. Support and hold objects by pressing the pelvis forward. A lack of lower body strength and stability, in combination with a lack of core strength, may have caused the pelvis to thrust forward in an attempt to find a comfortable position.

Breaking Bad Habits

We are creatures of habit. Not in terms of the things that make us feel safe or the things we like. But in the way we do things. Over time, we all create patterns in our bodies, and those patterns, if done often enough in one or two aspects of our lives, will show up in other areas.

Let's observe that Jim always walks and stands with his left foot turned outward. And then he decides he wants to lift weights or even start a yoga practice. And everything Jim does during those movements is with his left foot turned outward. Now unless someone catches that and points it out, his habit probably won't change.

But let's say Jim's yoga friend named Hope points this out, and Jim tries to change this position while performing an exercise. Upon practicing this exercise, he announces that his newly adapted foot position now hurts his knee, so he goes back to the way he was always doing it. The unfortunate consequence of this example is that Jim doesn't understand that his left foot turn-out is an adaptation. An adaptation to his environment, life in that environment of his truck, how he sits in it, how he lies in his bed, how he walks, even the shoes he wears, all encourage or discourage this pattern he has created.

With the right guidance and understanding of how the body moves and how his environment plays a role, Jim could instead work on that turn-out while he walks during the day, and he could pay attention and notice if he favors that left side or maybe leans when he sits in his truck seat. He can retrain his muscles to reflect healthier movement patterns (yes, a tiny turn-out can cause a slew of issues you never realized).

So instead of expecting a thirty-minute or sixty-minute exercise session to change a lifetime of adaptation, that exercise session can instead reaffirm, encourage, and feel out how things should be or can be in everyday life.

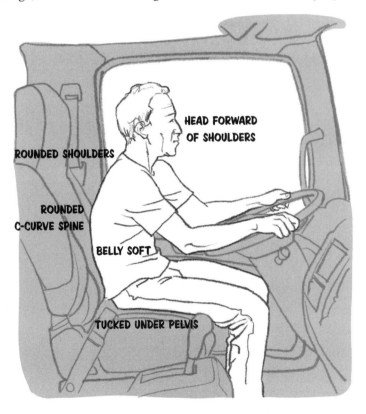

It may sound something like this: I wake up, get my clothes out, sit down to put them on. Then make or buy breakfast and sit down to eat my food. Then maybe walk to the bathroom to brush my teeth and walk to inspect my truck or collect my work items. Climb up into my truck and sit for the next several hours as I drive to my destination.

Somewhere along the way, I stop for a thirty-minute break where I go to the bathroom and then sit down and chill out for a few more minutes before I get back into my truck and sit some more. I drive to where I will park for the night. Get out of my vehicle, prepare dinner, or buy dinner, then sit down and eat, followed by a shower and then call it a night and sit or lie down and eventually sleep. This may happen in any order with a few details either missing or needing to be tweaked.

Your Daily Routine Check-In

Take a moment and think about how you do what you do each day—from the moment you wake up to the moment you go to sleep. Don't focus so much on what you are doing, but on how you do it.

From what you just read, how do you do what you do each day?

❑ How do you feel?

❑ What is your experience?

❑ Is it difficult to wake up, get out of bed?

❑ Do you struggle to get your socks, pants, or shoes on?

❑ Is getting in and out of your truck more difficult than it should be?

❑ Is all that sitting causing a pain in your neck or back?

❑ Do you always eat the same way?

❑ Drink the same way?

❑ Drive the same way?

❑ Stand or sit the same way?

It is critical to understand that how you do something is as important as what you are doing. Sure, you can get your shoes on, but is it a struggle? Is it optimal? Are you choosing to slide on your shoes so you don't have to bend down and tie them every day?

And if you are saying to yourself, "but I work out," please know that although that thirty to sixty minutes is excellent and will contribute to your ever-developing health journey, the reality is that going to the gym a few times a week hardly combats the daily twelve to eighteen hours you spent sitting with minimal movement.

The Rearview Mirror

We are a result of our environment over time. And as a truck driver, if being in the truck is not going to change, then it's time to change how you behave, move, and sit in the truck.

Rearview Mirror

Many drivers get into the driver's seat to start their day, sit upright, and often tilt the rearview mirror up to accommodate the alert posture. When you feel the temptation to adjust the mirror down, stop, and sit up taller instead. Adjust your body throughout the day, not your mirrors.

Behind-the-Wheel Posture

When you get behind the wheel, remember two important things: It's not your seat or steering wheel's responsibility to help you keep good posture. It's yours. Next time you get into the truck, check in to see what good posture would look and feel like before driving. Then ask yourself, "What do I need to do to keep it that way?" A small investment beforehand will save you a lifetime of pain and discomfort. Can you move the steering wheel? Can you adjust the seat? Can you get a seat support like a BackShield or an entirely new seat? Please don't wait until your posture is broken to fix it.

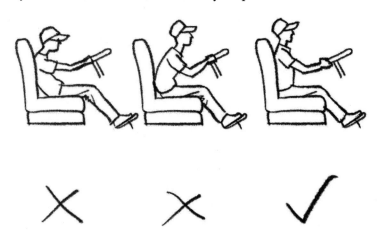

FIX YOUR POSTURE, FIX YOUR LIFE.
A DAILY POSTURE CHECK-IN CAN MAKE ALL THE DIFFERENCE IN HOW YOU FEEL.

4. 4 ESSENTIAL MOVES: BEND, REACH, ROTATE, AND SQUAT

Everyone must be able to age healthfully by bending, reaching, rotating, and squatting in the right way. When implemented correctly, these four moves become your everyday workout plan without even working out. They are your "stay in the life game plan," so you are not running old Betsy down the road on a prayer. Instead, you are roaring down the street with old Betsy like it was the first time out.

Everyone should be doing four basic movements: bending, reaching, rotating (sometimes called twisting), and squatting. We need to do them regularly, and we need to do them in a wide variety of ways to keep our bodies mobile and ready for the work environment and any elements that come our way. These moves are the key to a truck driver's well-being and for anyone who has a body and intends to use it throughout their lifetime.

As kids we naturally explored movement. We twisted and turned, bent and reached, squatted and rolled around without even thinking twice. And when our bodies gave us that itch to move, we moved. You don't need to be that kid lying upside down on the couch watching your favorite TV show, but you can take a cue from your younger self.

When I think of how our bodies need to move, I think about our joints. And when I think about our joints, I think about whether or not I am moving them, stretching them, and challenging their strength and mobility in as many ways as possible and at what frequency. The fact is our modern lives are cutting out one very important part of living—activity. And if you want to move when you get older, you best move now. Move frequently, move in various ways, at various heights, and carrying various loads. And when you are standing around, try to move instead of just standing.

At first adding in extra movements to my day felt a bit odd. I'm that person who cooks while I'm doing leg lifts and does laundry with the basket on the floor, making myself squat each time to pick up a new piece of clothing to fold. I always take the stairs and challenge myself to push it when I do. I park farther away and then challenge myself to carry my bags (if I don't have a million groceries) while trying to keep good posture. And by doing this, consciously putting movement into my day, guess what happened? I got stronger, my body hurt less, and I was happier, and when I moved more in my everyday life, exercise got easier.

A Note about Cardiovascular Exercise, Stretching, and Strength

These movement patterns can be tweaked and blinged out to your liking. Our bodies are dynamic and require other actions as well, such as cardiovascular activity to keep your heart strong. Find ways to get your heart rate up every single day. For example: Power walk around your truck, squat twenty times every time you go into the bathroom, hoof it up the stairs with a pep in your step.

Heart health is vital to our overall health and shouldn't be overlooked. One of the easiest ways to get your cardio in is walking. Walking at a brisk pace is an excellent way to help your heart. Walk the parking lot, park farther away at truck stops or grocery stores. Walk and talk on the phone, walk laps around your truck. It all adds up, and you'll have your health to show for it.

To keep our bodies healthy, mobile, and agile, stretching and strengthening must also be a part of the movement pie. Most people like to separate these two from each other, but really stretching and strengthening often happen at the same time.

What is stretching? Well stretching is what you can do to keep your muscles, ligaments, tendons, and fascia flexible and supple (think layers of tissues in different shapes, textures, sizes, thicknesses, and lengths). Our bodies need to be stretched daily if we want to freely use them. Use it or lose it could not be more true when it comes to our bodies. Without stretching, our muscles easily become short and tight and our fascia sticky, which leaves us immobile, stiff, and often in pain.

When you take a little time to stretch every day, you melt the build-up that is created, a layer that freezes over your tissues when you sleep at night. Just like rust that builds up when machine parts aren't used regularly and maintained properly, our bodies get build-up too. And the solution is to stretch and move.

Every time you lift your arm up overhead, you are stretching. Every time you squat down low, you are stretching. Every time you twist and turn, you are stretching. I want to encourage you to do these movements more and try to do them in new ways to push your boundaries. You will be amazed how much your body increases its range of movement and decreases its range of pain simply by stretching more throughout the day. Later, in this book, you will find a number of ways to stretch, and many of them can easily be added into your day.

Strengthening is another important aspect of movement. Why? Because without strength, how will you be able to carry your body from point A to point B, not to mention carry an object?

What is strengthening? I think of strengthening as improving muscle tone and mass, which often includes external forces or objects. When we work to strengthen our bodies, we can improve muscle mass and tone, increase bone density, which will help combat osteoporosis and improve bone health, as well as improve the overall strength of tendons and ligaments.

Our bodies are made up of a bunch of ropes and bungees that need to be stretched and strengthened regularly through various movements to keep our entire bodies happy and healthy. This book offers dozens of movements and exercises you can do throughout your day to both stretch and strengthen your body so that you can keep doing what you love and love doing it.

> *WARNING: Do not look at what you are about to read as "exercises."*
> *Look at the upcoming pages as a new way of living, moving, and being*
> *a trucker—life-enhancing moves you need to be doing every single day*
> *while living your life.*
> *YOUR ENVIRONMENT + EVERY MOVEMENT + YOU = FITNESS*

When you move forward with a mindset like that, you are already light-years ahead of where you were before.

Bending

If you want your joints to keep moving when you are in your seventies and beyond, you best keep moving them when you are in your forties, fifties, and sixties. Not all movement is created equal, and some activities are more prevalent than others in our daily lives.

Forward bending is a primary everyday function we all do to keep our lives moving. On average, in twenty hours, including sleeping, we bend over 2,000 to 4,000 times a day. Except most of this bending we do is ill postured and hurting us more than helping us.

As a truck driver, all that sitting, coupled with a seat that offers no support or reduced impact, leaves a driver with back pain every day. When you look out across other cultures worldwide, few struggle with back pain like we do in the West, and it all boils down to one important concept: they have good posture.

Rounding versus Bending

Rounding your body is not the same as bending your body, explicitly bending forward. But when you spend most of your day in a rounded or hunched position, either sitting or standing, that will carry over into your other daily movements and habits. Several years into teaching yoga, I saw a gap in my teaching, and I wanted to fix that. I knew postures, I knew people in those postures, but I didn't know people, I didn't know the movements that those people were doing and should be making, and I wanted to fix that.

Each of your body parts plays a specific role in how you move. Next time you need to reach down and pick up something, remember your hip hinges the body like a hinge on a door. The door doesn't bend in the middle, and neither should you. If your hinge is tight or restricted (hamstring, hip, or back tightness), simply bend the knees to help you get safely further.

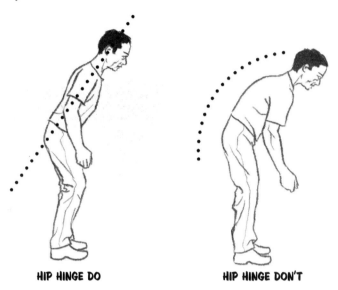

HIP HINGE DO   **HIP HINGE DON'T**

Now ask yourself, how many times a day are you bending forward? How many of those times are you bending effectively?

Not all bending is created equal and done equally efficiently. When you bend, you want to think of bending at a joint, like a hinge on your truck door. A door doesn't bend in the middle. A door moves at its hinge point, and the same goes for your body. Doing so will reduce the chance of injury and request all the surrounding body parts to participate. This is a short book, and I want to explain all the ways to bend and improve your bendability, and I think the best way to do that is with pictures.

Bending toward a Better Body Check-In

Forward bending happens regularly in our daily lives, but not all forward bends are created equal. Let's take inventory of how it is you bend to improve how your body feels.

A forward bend happens at three main points: the hip joint, the pelvis and sacrum, and the lower lumbar.

Try this:

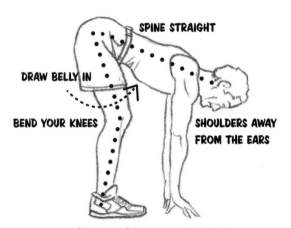

SPINE STRAIGHT

DRAW BELLY IN

BEND YOUR KNEES

SHOULDERS AWAY FROM THE EARS

SHIFT WEIGHT FORWARD IN FEET

Forward Bend

Now ask yourself the following questions:

❏ How does this feel?

❏ What feels tight? Calves? Hamstrings? Lower back? Upper back? Neck?

❏ What feels mobile or moves easily?

❏ Is one side tighter than the other?

❏ Does your body enjoy the experience, or is it fighting it?

❏ When you rise back up, do you feel stiff? Or are you relieved and open?

When you add more effective forward bending into your day, you can help your body age healthfully and move about more productively.

Lifting

The next time you drop something on the ground, remember to bend and squat. This effective practice will eliminate strains and pains in the back by shifting the load to your hips, glutes, and legs, rather than to your lower back.

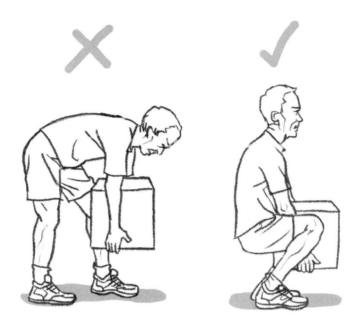

PROPER LIFTING CAN MAKE ALL THE DIFFERENCE IN HOW YOUR BODY FEELS. WHEN LIFTING HEAVY OBJECTS, REMEMBER TO ENGAGE YOUR GLUTES MUSCLES, KEEP YOUR HIPS UNDERNEATH YOU, AND STAY UPRIGHT.

For the next twenty-four hours, notice when your day presents an opportunity to insert a quick forward bend. When do you have dead air time? A gap or space to do something, and instead, you are just standing or sitting there? These could be moments while you are filling up the tank with fuel, or in the bathroom stall, or while sitting or standing around talking on the phone.

Assess where you are bending and ask yourself if you could be using better mechanics. Are you hunching over to pick up your shoe? Are you hunching forward to pick up a dropped tool? Are you striking a pose and doing a forward bend to stretch your back and hamstrings, but instead of taking a quick second to set up your body, are you throwing yourself into the pose? These movements don't take a lot of time. But when you start to draw awareness to them, little by little, you can alter how you feel in your body and your life.

Ways to Bend

Here are a few of my favorite forward bends to help you along the way.

STANDING

- Straight leg hip hinge: Stand tall and point your toes forward. Place your hands on your hips and fold only as far as you can without bending your knees or rounding your spine. Lean into your toes slightly to feel the stretch.
- Bent-knee hip hinge: Stand tall and point your toes forward. Place your hands at your hips and bend your knees. Fold only as far as you can without rounding your spine. If necessary, place your hands on a chair or step.
- One knee down forward bend: Stand tall and step one foot back. Slowly begin to bend both knees and drop your back knee to the ground and bend forward.
- Straddle forward bend: Step your feet wide into a legs length position and turn your toes forward. Place your hands at your hips or on a stool, step, or table in front of you. Slowly hinge from your hips and bend as far as you can forward toward the ground. Lean gently into your toes to increase the stretch.

SEATED

- Bent-knee forward bend: Seated, bend both knees in front of you and place a pillow under your legs. Slowly tip your torso forward to lie over your thighs and reach for your toes with your hands or a strap.
- Seated straddle: Seated, widen your legs (bend your knees if your hamstrings are tight) and with a long spine slowly lean forward from your hips. Walk your hands out in front of you and reach to stretch your spine.
- Chair forward bend: Seated at the edge of a chair widen your legs to a position wider than the chair's width. Slowly hinge forward from your hips and lower your torso toward the mouth of the chair letting your arms hang toward the ground.

LYING DOWN

- Legs up the wall: Sit with your hip and side up next to the wall. Slowly lie down as you spin your legs up the wall. Relax your spine and, if necessary, support your head. Extend your arms overhead to rest alongside your ears.
- Straddle legs up the wall: Repeat the previous move, but this time allow your legs to slide wide down the wall.

Reaching

Over an entire day, how many times do you reach up? Grab something overhead? Lift your arms above your shoulders for any reason? Truck driver or not, most of us don't do it enough. And as we age, for fear of getting hurt, we remove the items and actions from our lives that require us to reach up overhead, and we eliminate the things and actions from our day that require us to squat down. We stop performing these actions for the sake of convenience, time, and health.

But reaching is a necessary function of living healthy. Sure, let's not pull down on hefty doors or reach for tools that weigh hundreds of pounds that might fall on our heads. But the action of reaching is not something you should eliminate from your life, no matter what age and what profession you come from.

Put Your Hands in the Air

The simple act of reaching your arms up overhead is a full-body action. Think of your arm like the shifter in the truck; when you shift gears, the truck moves. When you move your arms, your body responds. I tell all my students that your arms are an extension of your core and back. Everything is connected. When we feel stiffness in our lower back, I often look to the arms' use and range of motion.

Latissimus Dorsi Muscle

The latissimus dorsi is our largest back muscle and connects our pelvis and lower back to our arms. Reach up with your arms, and you are stretching your lower back. Never reach with your arms, and your lower back will never get the movement it deserves and requires.

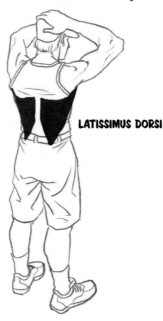

LATISSIMUS DORSI

The arm itself (humorous bone) serves as the attachment site for the latissimus dorsi muscle, which means when you don't reach your arms up overhead, your back suffers. Think of it as a pulley system. Lift arms, stretch back. Don't lift arms, don't stretch back.

Most people think about bending forward when it comes to stretching the back. But that isn't the only way.

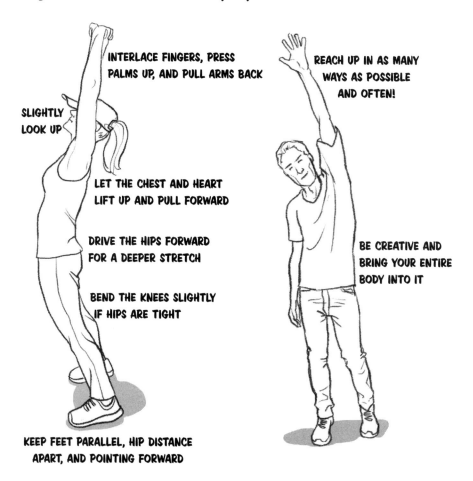

INTERLACE FINGERS, PRESS PALMS UP, AND PULL ARMS BACK

SLIGHTLY LOOK UP

REACH UP IN AS MANY WAYS AS POSSIBLE AND OFTEN!

LET THE CHEST AND HEART LIFT UP AND PULL FORWARD

DRIVE THE HIPS FORWARD FOR A DEEPER STRETCH

BE CREATIVE AND BRING YOUR ENTIRE BODY INTO IT

BEND THE KNEES SLIGHTLY IF HIPS ARE TIGHT

KEEP FEET PARALLEL, HIP DISTANCE APART, AND POINTING FORWARD

When you reach up overhead, you open tight shoulders, improve posture, and strengthen and improve arm and shoulder strength. You also reduce and prevent back pain, reduce fatigue, and even improve leg function by increasing circulation. The best part is, you can do this anytime, anywhere. And you can start today, right from the cab of your truck.

Raise Your Hands in the Air Check-In

☐ Think about your current life. What do you do each day, and what could you do each day? Take inventory of this one action—reaching—and how frequently it's performed.

☐ How many times a day do you reach your arms up above your shoulders?

☐ How many of those reaching actions do you do because your daily life requires them?

☐ How many of those actions are performed because you inserted that action into your day on purpose?

☐ How far can you reach overhead?

☐ How far can you reach overhead without allowing your chest and front ribs to lift up?

Reaching is a primary life movement, not an exercise.

Reaching
Conveniently, our daily lives makes it less and less necessary to reach up and grab something, so reach up and stretch as many times as you can throughout the day. Make sure you reach up every time you get up from your seat.

Ways to Reach

☐ Reach up with one arm overhead.

☐ Reach up with both arms overhead.

☐ Reach up while holding a gallon of water, tool, or hand weight.

☐ Reach up and hang (think monkey bars).

☐ Reach up and side bend.

☐ Stand with arms against the wall in a cactus position. Do your head, back, and arms touch the wall?

☐ Reach up and bend backward.

☐ Wave.

☐ Do arm circles.

☐ Reach up and pretend to pick cherries overhead.

☐ Perform a triceps stretch.

☐ Stretch in bed.

Reach However You Can

Put your hands in the air, like you just don't care. How many ways can you think of reaching your arms up and overhead? Next time you are just standing around, stand around with your arms up away from the ground.

Get your hands up. Reach up. Notice how infrequently you reach your arms above your shoulders. Let's start a new trend: random reach-ups. And put your whole body into it. So now reaching for that cup in the high cabinet is a full-body experience.

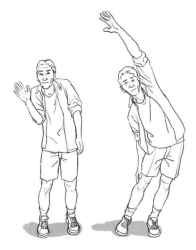

PAY ATTENTION TO HOW OFTEN YOU DON'T REACH OVERHEAD AND HOW OFTEN YOUR ARMS DON'T FULLY EXTEND. TRY TO INCORPORATE MORE REACHING INTO YOUR DAY IN ALL DIFFERENT WAYS AND GET YOUR ENTIRE BODY INVOLVED.

Seated Reaching

During those many downtimes while driving, put your arms into it. Reach up, reach back, reach around, and keep moving. Driving doesn't have to be done just while sitting if you don't let it.

Don't wait until you are at a sports game to put your arms up in the air. Finding those little pockets of time is simple. In the next twenty-four hours, set your alarm at one-hour intervals. When the alarm goes off, find as many ways to reach your arms up overhead as possible. Reach your arms to the side, on an angle, behind you. Anywhere you can. And if you are like me and try to get in as many steps a day as possible, change it up.

When you are walking, do arm circles, reach up like you are picking apples, add a set of light hand-weights and press up overhead and in as many directions as you can. The name of the game is use it or lose it. If you want to keep using your arms, you need to start using them in as many ways as possible, including reaching up overhead.

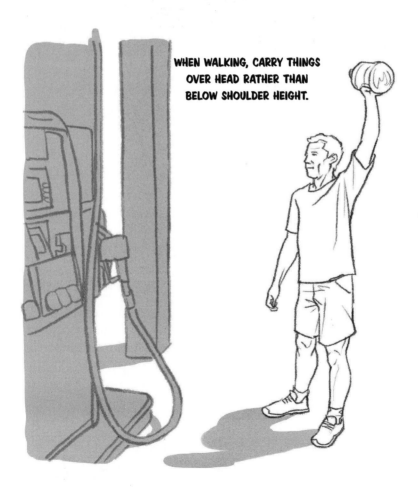

WHEN WALKING, CARRY THINGS OVER HEAD RATHER THAN BELOW SHOULDER HEIGHT.

Rotating

The swivel chair is the best worst invention of our time. It may make working in your office, moving from desk to desk, or sliding onto a stool at a table and talking between the two people on either side of you much more comfortable. However, it doesn't make your body any healthier. Instead of you rotating, the chair now does it for you.

Stability, Mobility, and Strength

Rotation offers our bodies a fantastic opportunity for a combination of experiences—one that squatting and bending don't necessarily provide. When you rotate your entire body, you need all three of these to occur: stability, mobility, and strength. Activities like throwing, kicking, swinging, pulling, even pushing all require rotation.

Why am I talking about rotating and not twisting? Well, twisting is often directed toward a spinal movement, where rotation can be a complete body action, one that requests more of your body and joints to get involved. Try this: Look over your shoulder, notice what happens. Now look over your shoulder and keep turning, not just at the neck but let that movement trickle down your entire body. The next time you look over your shoulder, rotate your body, and if you pay close attention, you should notice your entire spine getting involved, down to your hips and ankles. Let this serve as a gateway for you to find other opportunities to add rotation into your life. You should focus on places where you are already rotating, but could explore in more depth, or areas where you aren't and should or could be. You have to start somewhere, so let that somewhere be here.

As a truck driver, you probably spend little time on a swivel office chair, but even as a driver in a forward facing driver's seat, your mobility is significantly reduced by the amount of rotating you do throughout the day. Your semi-truck may not have a backup camera. Still, your regular ride may, and that backup camera, although it can help you squeeze into the parking space on a dime or line up your pickup and trailer with ease, has robbed you of another opportunity to rotate.

Twist and Shout

When you rotate, you turn, revolving, twisting, ringing out the towel of your body, and often the focus is the spine. But you can also rotate your hips and shoulders, your ankles, and wrists, too. Rotation is frequently described as a joint movement, and if you want your joints to stay healthy, strong, and mobile, you need to rotate them.

Without rotation in our everyday lives, our bodies suffer. Rotation nourishes the disks between our vertebrae and keeps the tissues in our bodies supple, and rotation at our joints helps our joint capsules stay lubricated.

I challenge you to find all the ways you can twist and turn your body when you wouldn't otherwise. When you grab your seatbelt, reach for it with your outside arm and exaggerate the twist and click. Just while sitting around, add a little torso rotation. Roll your wrists and ankles regularly.

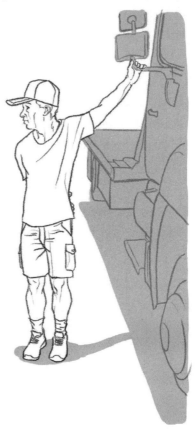

GRAB SOMETHING AND ROTATE.

WHEN YOU START TO TWIST YOUR BODY, PRACTICE TURNING TOWARDS THE OBJECT (TRUCK) AND AWAY FROM IT. NOTICE HOW EACH MOVEMENT FEELS. HERE HE'S ROTATING HIS BODY AWAY FROM THE TRUCK FOR A GREAT HIP, TRUNK, AND CHEST STRETCH.

Caution: Rotate Slowly

I have watched thousands of people rotate their bodies, and one thing I have noticed is the aggressive nature that can often accompany this movement. And the problem with an approach like this is you end up overstretching or twisting the areas that are already mobile and neglecting the areas that need the movement.

Take the spine, for example. If you are mobile in the neck and upper torso (spine), but not the lower back and hip area, then when you twist in a yoga class or everyday life, that movement will more than likely be exaggerated in the areas that move well. And as for the areas that don't move very well, they will be skipped. The same can be correct for the right and left sides of our bodies. Daily movement patterns, our jobs, and even where things are located (in the cab of the truck, for example) can leave us rotating more to one side than the other.

When they notice areas of imbalance in strength, stability, rotation, and mobility, I tell my students to use the 2:1 ratio. If you can rotate easily to the right but not to the left, increase the amount of movement on the weaker, tighter, or stiffer side. You can easily take this approach on the yoga mat and in life. This might mean vacuuming with your left hand instead of your right. Or when you go to click your seatbelt, pretending to do the same to the other side and holding that stretch. Remember, it's the little things that add up over time.

That type of approach to rotation can leave your body imbalanced and in pain and lead to a greater risk of injury. Instead of trying to go deeper in your rotations and twists, try to move the restricted areas instead. Your ego may not like it as much, but you will see more significant strides in how your body moves in all that you do.

Tummy Troubles

Twisting helps your muscles, and, at the same time, twisting your torso can often improve digestion and elimination and reduce flatulence (the fancy word for gas). All that stretching, compressing, and contracting can also increase blood flow to various body areas. And for those of us who are stagnant during the day, that added burst of blood flow can be just what our body ordered.

When we twist the torso (our spine), we compress (massage) our internal organs and bring more blood flow to them. If your digestion is less than ideal, is it the food you are eating, or is it that your body isn't moving enough to help digest it?

I don't want to get in the weeds here, as this book is about movement, but my point is that our bodies are meant to move, and when we move in various ways, that movement helps our bodies in multiple ways. By adding in a simple spinal twist, you can reduce back pain and improve digestion and elimination.

Try lying down on your back in your sleeper before you go to bed and draw your leg across your body in a twist and then repeat on the other side. Your back and tummy will be happy you did. Sounds like a great two-for-one special if I ever heard one.

WELLNESS PITSTOP CHECKLIST

Body Rotation Check-In

- ❑ Take inventory of your daily to do list. Take inventory of what types of movements are required for you to do them. Do any of them require you to rotate?

- ❑ Where in your day could you rotate more? Where are you only going halfway (think about the seatbelt example)? And where can you move more?

- ❑ Think about which directions you rotate during the day. Do you rotate more to the right than the left?

- ❑ How can you change that?

- ❑ When you turn your head, do you go as far as you can go? Or just far enough to get the job done?

- ❑ When you turn your torso, do you maximize that opportunity and get your entire torso and spine involved or do you go just far enough to get the job done?

☐ Stand or sit tall and move your arms up and overhead in a circle forward and back. How do they move? How do they not move?

☐ When you throw, swing, kick, push, or pull, how can you bring more of your body into the movement?

☐ When you rotate, what moves easily and what doesn't?

☐ Stand and turn your shoulders and not your hips, then reverse it. Which is easier, what pulls, what feels tight, and what feels mobile?

☐ When you lift or lower your landing gear on your trailer, do you just use your shoulder or your whole body?

Types of Rotation

☐ Turn your head and look over your shoulder as far as you can.

☐ Rotate (twist) your torso at the belly, rib cage, shoulders, and neck.

☐ While standing, turn and twist your hips right and left.

☐ Rotate your ankles.

☐ Rotate your wrists.

☐ Plant one foot and rotate your entire body from the ground up by lifting the opposite foot and twisting.

☐ Throw a ball, bringing your entire body through the motions of the wind-up and release.

☐ Push or pull something and work to use your entire body, not just your arms.

☐ Rotate to the right and then the left and notice which of your sides is more mobile.

☐ Rotate your arms in a circle at the shoulder joint.

☐ Rotate your legs in a circle at the hip joint.

Don't just rotate your tires, rotate your body, too. Now that you are aware of this movement pattern called rotation, notice how seldom you may be doing it, and furthermore how little of the actual movement you are taking advantage of.

To me, rotation creates relief—relief from tension, relief from restriction, relief from tightness that shouldn't be there. Rotation liberates the body. Commit one entire day to finding all the pockets of time where you can purposefully add rotation into your routine and notice when you are rotating your body so you can challenge yourself to go further.

Squatting

Earlier in my life I lived in Nigeria. I worked at an orphanage and stayed with a family in Ibadan, Nigeria. Nigeria was a third world country, and their lifestyle differed vastly from ours. This began with the uneven roads and walk-ways. Thousands of people walked to their destinations and carried their bags, items, kids, and water.

As I walked through the streets, it was not uncommon to see patrons squatting at their table while eating their food. And most public bathrooms were holes in the ground—some very nice ones. But if I had to go, it was a good thing I could squat low. Some in our modern world call it a more challenging life. But is it? Is it a harder life?

You want to be a forklift, not a crane.

Forklift

When you squat, it is necessary that you don't just focus on how you go down, but how you come back up, too. When you come up, you want to be powered from underneath by the forklift: your glutes, your core, pelvic floor, and hamstrings. By squatting your hips back and powering up from underneath, you get a more powerful workout and a more balanced backside.

Crane

When you squat, make sure you aren't powered by the crane when you come back up. Lifting your head first unnecessarily uses your back and quad muscles and leaves your core, glutes, and hamstrings out of the equation. You not only lose out on proper muscle building, but moving in such a way can lead to serious injury. Next time you come up from a squat, make sure the forklift is lifting you, not the crane.

When you squat, you do a lot for your body. When you squat regularly in various ways, no matter the environment, your body benefits. The long-term effects of sitting have made it more challenging to squat correctly. When your calves become short and tight, your glutes and hamstrings don't fire as needed, so your squat acts more like a crane than a forklift. Let me explain.

When you squat and your body weight shifts forward into your toes and knees, not only is that hard on your knees, but your quadriceps (thigh muscles) are more likely to fire and be the muscles to get the job done. When your calves are mobile and unrestricted, glutes and hamstrings fire properly, and when you squat down, then you can use the forklift to get back upright. Why does this matter? It matters because your body frequently requires balance—front to back, top to bottom, right to left. And when you sit all day on the back side of your body, you suffer.

It appears the older you get, the more afraid you are of squatting. Except squatting is a fundamental movement pattern you have been doing since you were a baby. And as you get older, you have slowly stopped these basic and necessary movement patterns due to convenience, work requirements, and dare I say, laziness. I mean, why would you if you don't have to? My response to that is, you may not need to do it now, but by leaving out these movements, you may come to find that there is a trickle effect, and other areas of your life will be affected.

Bathroom Behavior

Why squat and poo like I did in Nigeria? Squatting while toileting can help you empty your bowels more efficiently. The inside of your body is much like a map, with roads leading to all sorts of destinations. And when one road appears to be blocked, it can stall the objects moving along it—in this case, poop. The positions we put our bodies in can either block off a road or open it up. The long-term effects of sitting in today's world come with negative consequences.

I giggle because the invention of the Squatty Potty is not new (see the website for a photo at www.SquattyPotty.com). It's merely a plastic step that lifts your feet so that when you sit on your porcelain throne, the step positions your body much like it should be situated when it's time to go and still is in many countries across the globe.

Furthermore, as you age, the negative consequences of straining while you go can have unfortunate effects on your body's other areas, such as your heart. You may want to fight me on this technique. But I assure you a simple change, such as lifting your feet while you hit the loo, could be the magic solution to all your pooping problems.

Squat

Some people have the mobility to squat but not the strength; others can squat but don't have the mobility to get low. When squatting, pay attention to how far you can go before your pelvis wants to tuck or drop forward. That's the end of your healthy range. Help your squat by holding a chair or pole, reach up for a countertop or a step, and hold on. And keep at it; each day, your technique will get better and better.

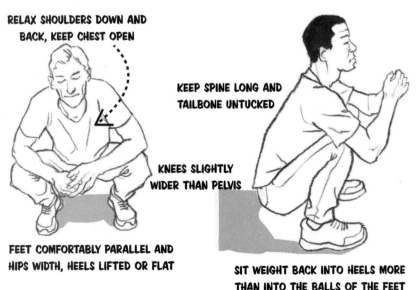

RELAX SHOULDERS DOWN AND BACK, KEEP CHEST OPEN

KEEP SPINE LONG AND TAILBONE UNTUCKED

KNEES SLIGHTLY WIDER THAN PELVIS

FEET COMFORTABLY PARALLEL AND HIPS WIDTH, HEELS LIFTED OR FLAT

SIT WEIGHT BACK INTO HEELS MORE THAN INTO THE BALLS OF THE FEET

It's Not the Squat's Fault

Are squats bad? Some say they are hard on the knees, while others say their body isn't made to squat. What if it's not that your body can't squat, but instead has adopted a life void of squatting that has now made it difficult to do so? Is it that squatting wrecks the knees or that not squatting over an extended period has put a strain on your knees, so now when you desire to do so it is difficult?

Human beings like yourself all over the world squat. Right now, this very second, someone is squatting, not because they are in a yoga class, but because they see it as a movement beneficial for their daily life. They've squatted to tie their shoe. They have squatted to pick up a pen on the ground. They have squatted because their back is feeling stiff, and they need to move. You can be that person.

It is my opinion that we have merely unlearned these essential functions. And the good news is we can relearn them starting today. Squats may not be as easy as they once were when you were a small child or in your twenties or forties, but you can most definitely do them. Try these movements to improve your ability to squat:

KNEES TO CHEST

The knees to chest lying down squat is a perfect version for those who feel strain while squatting upright.

- Lie on your back. Bring your knees into your chest and grab hold of your shins or hamstrings or, if necessary, use a belt and drape it over your shins and grab hold.
- Exhale and compress your thighs to your belly.
- Work to unroll your tailbone out onto the bed or floor and lengthen your spine.
- Relax your shoulders and breathe.

KNEELING SQUAT—ALSO CALLED THE CHILD'S POSE (SEE CHAPTER 6, SLEEPER POSES)

This is another version of a squat done while kneeling. It's great for relaxation, and the arm extension is an added bonus.

- Start on all fours. Exhale and start to sit back as far as your body will allow trying to keep your pelvis from tucking under.
- Spread the knees wider if necessary and make room for your chest and middle.
- Slide the arms farther forward and reach through your fingertips to create a stretch from tailbone to fingertips.
- Rest the head on a pillow if necessary.

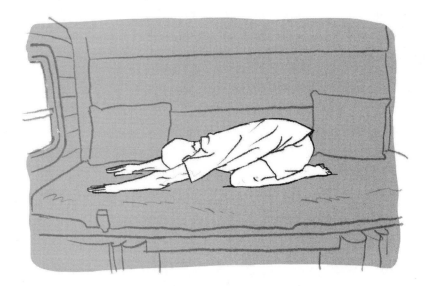

SQUATTING DOESN'T JUST HAVE TO BE FROM A STANDING POSITION. EASE YOUR BODY INTO A SQUAT BY TRYING THIS POSITION IN A KNEELING POSITION OR ON YOUR BACK.

Do You Know Squat Check-In

There are lots of ways to squat. So if one doesn't work for you right now, try another. But see if you can find as many opportunities throughout your day to add in a few squats here and there. Standing around refueling? Squat. In the bathroom stall? Sneak in ten squats. Before you put on your pants for the day? Squat. Lying in bed? Squat. Use the following list as a reference to help you add more types of squats to your life. Don't wait for that exercise class to do so; you can start now.

P.S.: Use support. (Don't be embarrassed or decide not to do it because you can't. How will you ever teach your body if you won't even try?)

Squatting is a primary life movement, not an exercise.

Types of Squats

PREPARATION SQUATS

These are the movements to get your body ready for squatting, so if you can't squat now, don't worry, start here.

- Table squat with toes unrolled: Come down onto your hands and knees. With your toes unrolled begin to lean back toward your heels a few inches to increase the stretch.
- Table squat with toes curled under: Come down onto your hands and knees. With your shoes off, try to curl your toes under and, if able, begin to lean back toward your heels a few inches to increase the stretch.
- Rocking squat: Come down onto your hands and knees. Keep your belly strong, and as you exhale, slowly rock back toward

your heels as far as you can go. Inhale and rise back up to all fours. Repeat this five to ten times.

- Bed squat (lying on bed): Lie down on your back, place your hands behind your thighs or knees (or loop a strap or belt behind your thigh if you cannot reach). Gently begin to draw your legs in toward your body. Allow the legs to come wide and let your knees drop towards the bed (imagine you are squatting on the ceiling).

- Calf stretch: Standing tall with your 5-Point Posture in check, take a casual step back with one foot. Point both feet forward. Slightly bend the front knee and freeze it in place. As you exhale, bend the back knee without lifting the heel. Repeat five to ten times on each side.

SQUATS

- High squat: Step your feet open to a wide stance. Turn your toes slightly out and bend your knees to sit over your ankles. Keep your body upright and tall.

- Functional squat: Step your feet open to a wide stance. Keep your feet parallel, and as you bend your knees, push your hips back and lean your torso forward (imagine your back on a coffee table). And try reaching your arms forward alongside your ears and stretch your tailbone to your fingertips.

- Chair hovering squat: Take a seat at the edge of a chair. Step your feet hip distance apart (or closer) and point your toes forward. Lift yourself off your chair and hover one to two inches above the seat. Try to reach your arms alongside your ears or raise them like a cactus. Draw your belly in and keep your spine long.

- Deep/yogic squat: Step your feet hip distance apart. If necessary allow your toes a slight turn out. Slowly lower yourself down as far as you can go. Notice at what point your heels want to lift (if this happens, see the Calf Stretch Prep Squat).

- Assisted squat: If you struggle to get down in your deep squat, try this move. Grab a pole, sturdy chair leg, or table leg and lower yourself down into a squat. Fully extend your arms and lean back into your hips and heels.
- Low heel squat: Step your feet hip distance (or slightly wider) apart and point your toes forward. Bend your knees and lower down. Allow your heels to lift and let your knees come apart. Drop your torso between your knees and reach forward. As you do so, lean back into your hips and heels.
- One-legged kneeling squat: Start in a split stance, one foot back. Slowly bend the back knee and lower to the ground and set your back knee on the ground near the ankle of your front leg. Use support to get down and up if needed.

Find one to three types of squats or preparation movements for squats from the previous list that you can do. It doesn't have to be pretty, but choose a few that you can commit to. And three times a day for the next week, insert these movements into your day on purpose.

Suppose something drops, squat to pick it up. If you are standing around before you have to hop in the truck, squat for five breaths. Ask yourself where in your day you can consciously add squatting.

In the beginning, you can start by just hugging your knees into your chest while lying in bed on your back. Or if you are sitting on the bottom step of your truck, open your legs and lean forward a bit. Or maybe you buy a Squatty Potty for your bathroom at home so you can squat and go. We all have to start somewhere. And as these movements become more automatic, they will become a part of your everyday life, like brushing your teeth or putting on your shoes.

PART II

IN-CAB FITNESS:
GET FIT WHILE YOU SIT

I f you've gotten this far, you know the key to improving your physical and mental health is initiating more movement throughout your day. Once I started exploring basic movement, it amazed me how simple it can be to insert more movement into activities we do every day.

Today, I challenge you to look at your environment and see opportunities to participate actively in your life. You might feel silly or uncomfortable at first. We all feel that way at times when doing something new.

In this second part of the book, I show you moves that you can do in the driver's seat, the sleeper, and outside your truck that will improve the way you feel. When to insert these moves into your day is up to you.

When I see a chair, a bench, a truck step, a pole, a bathroom stall, or an elevator, I see opportunities to move and exercise. And you'll see other opportunities, too. When you wake up, can you stretch at the edge of your bed? When you reach down to grab your shoe, can you turn that into a squat? While you are driving, sitting, or standing around, can you move in any way?

If you take my advice, by the end of the day, you will have added five, fifteen, even forty-five minutes of extra movement that you wouldn't have had otherwise. Not to mention if you park farther away at rest stops and walk more... Heck, I might even spot you in the fitness center at a truck stop or striking a yoga pose outside your truck. That extra movement adds up, and you will reap the rewards of feeling better, wherever you are—in the truck, a parking lot, or at home. You'll age healthier and help stave off preventable chronic illness. You, my friend, win!

CAUTION: The following are suggestions to improve your physical health as a truck driver. At no point does this book or the exercises in it suggest that drivers should jeopardize the safety of their driving to participate in any of the following movements. Please use common sense while driving and while performing any of the exercises described below.

Each of these moves can be done individually throughout the day or be put together to create a mini exercise routine. It is not necessary to do all the exercises listed each day—rather, commit to adding in one to five moves until they become automatic, and then slowly add in a few more.

It is vital to understand that following the guidance of this book may result in reduced pain, a more active life, and an increase in happiness.

5. YOU IN THE DRIVER'S SEAT

You may be stuck all day or night in the driver's seat because that is what your job requires you to do. But that seat you sit in day in and day out has more than one purpose. It is your job to find ways, times, and places to get moving. And what better place than in the seat of your truck?

It might seem awkward at first, but I assure you, once you get moving, you will feel the effects of reaching, twisting, extending, and bending. Don't wait until your day is over and you are free from your truck seat to get up and move. Think of the necessity to sit for hours as an opportunity created just for you to do any of the following moves.

And when you aren't in the truck, find a chair, use your couch, or find a bench. There are pockets of time everywhere, and once you are aware of them, you can take advantage of them. Have fun with these moves; challenge yourself to do a few each day. Chances are if you are reading this book then you have been looking for ways to get moving more, exercise more, and improve your health. All that's left is to get moving.

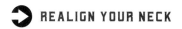

NECK STRETCH

The neck stretch counterbalances the forward head position and tightness you get from hunching forward over the steering wheel.

- Sit tall with your feet on the floor in the driver's seat.
- Relax your shoulders. Open your mouth.
- Drop your head back.
- Close your mouth and press your bottom jaw and chin to the sky.
- Slide your bottom jaw side to side.
- Do this for 5 to 10 breaths.
- For best results, repeat 2 to 4 times a day.

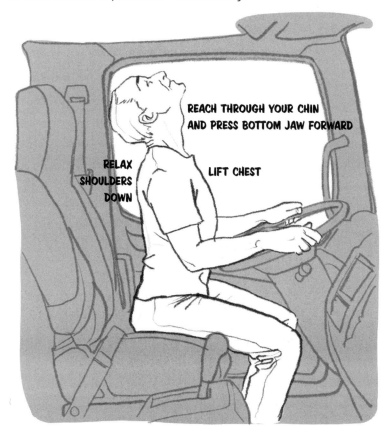

REACH THROUGH YOUR CHIN AND PRESS BOTTOM JAW FORWARD

RELAX SHOULDERS DOWN

LIFT CHEST

NERVE GLIDES

Reduce the tension accumulated in your neck and shoulders from driving or computer work.

- Sit tall with feet flat on the ground.
- Relax your shoulders down.
- Drop your left arm down and flex your palm (facing down).
- Place your right hand on the left side of your head above your ear.
- Tip your head to the left.
- Gently draw down on the side of your head with your hand.
- Continue to press on the seat with the heel of your left hand, creating space between your shoulder and ear.
- Hold this for 5 to 10 breaths.
- Repeat on the other side.

Do in the driver's seat, in a chair, or standing around when you notice neck pain

....

Move head and hand around to change the stretch

....

Do this at least once a day to help combat neck pain

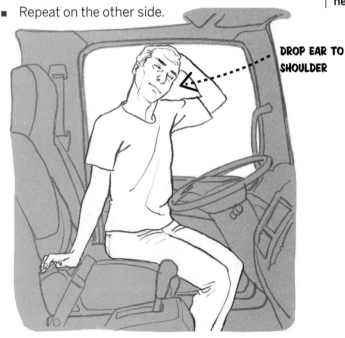

DROP EAR TO SHOULDER

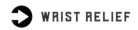

VISOR WRIST STRETCH

Wrist and carpal tunnel issues can be a side-effect of gripping and repetitive strain. Give your wrists and forearms a little relief.

- Sit tall in the driver's seat.
- Extend your arms up toward the visor (or steering wheel).
- Externally rotate your arms, turning the folds of the elbows up.
- Place your hands onto the visor and press into the heels of your hands.
- Hold this for 5 breaths.

Repeat 2 to 4 times per day

....

Do this when waiting to load or unload

....

Try this against the steering wheel

....

Try this by pulling back on your fingers with your opposite hand

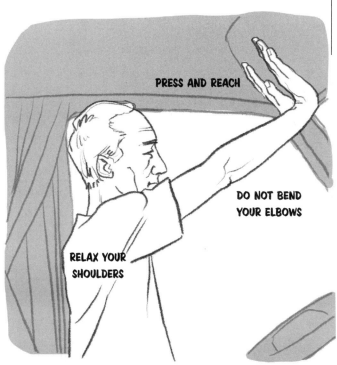

PRESS AND REACH

DO NOT BEND YOUR ELBOWS

RELAX YOUR SHOULDERS

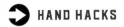
STEERING WHEEL HAND STRETCHES

Reduce pain and strain from gripping the steering wheel where your hands are in constant flexion.

- Take one hand and hang your thumb off the edge of the steering wheel.
- Press your hand down as you keep your thumb secure on the wheel.
- Hold that stretch for 10 seconds.
- Repeat the same process and work through each finger.
- Repeat on the opposite hand and repeat daily 2 to 6 times a day.

Try this stretch against the steering wheel, side of a table or against the side of your truck

....

Try stretching all your fingertips at the same time

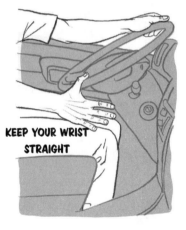

KEEP YOUR WRIST STRAIGHT

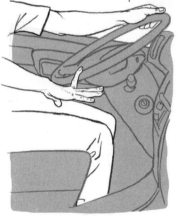

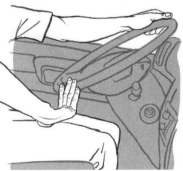

OPEN YOUR ENTIRE HAND AND LENGTHEN THROUGH YOUR FINGERTIPS

DRIVER'S SEAT ARM STRETCHES

Moving your arms regularly is critical to your physical health. Keep your upper body open and mobile while driving.

- Sit tall in the driver's seat.
- Take one arm and reach it up toward the ceiling above you and stretch your arm.
- Next, take that same arm and stretch it out to the side, grab hold of the passenger seat, and stretch.
- Finally, tuck your arm behind you and draw back on your elbow to open the shoulder.
- Hold each position for 5 to 10 breaths each.
- Repeat this sequence 2 to 4 times per day.

You may need to get a bit more creative on the opposite side

....

If your location allows it, roll down your window and stretch your arm out to the side

....

Get creative. How many other ways can you stretch your arms?

....

When reaching your arm up overhead find something to grab onto and then relax your body to stretch even more

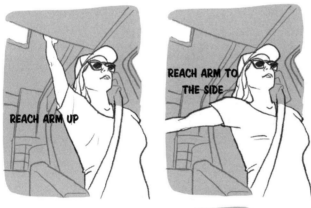

REACH ARM UP

REACH ARM TO THE SIDE

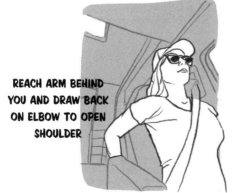

REACH ARM BEHIND YOU AND DRAW BACK ON ELBOW TO OPEN SHOULDER

DRIVER'S SEAT HEADREST CHEST OPENER

The long-term effects of sitting and driving can cause hunching and upper back and neck strain. Use this stretch to combat those challenges.

- Place both feet flat on the floor.
- Sit tall and lean back against the seat.
- Take both of your hands and reach back for the headrest.
- Press your palms against the headrest and at the same time press your elbows back and open.
- Hold for 5 to 10 breaths.
- Repeat 2 to 4 times daily.

If your hands are unable to touch the headrest, grab a belt or sock and walk your hands together as close as possible

....

Feel your chest open and shoulder blades come together

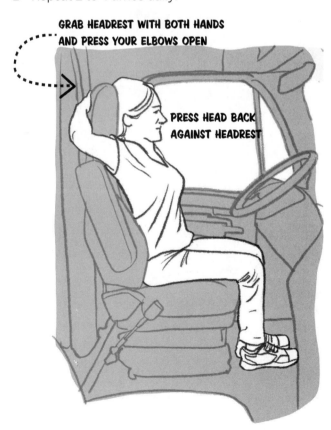

GRAB HEADREST WITH BOTH HANDS AND PRESS YOUR ELBOWS OPEN

PRESS HEAD BACK AGAINST HEADREST

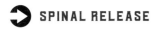

SEAT BELT TWIST

Ring out the sponge that is your spine with a quick twist. Rotation can relieve your back of tension, tightness, and strain.

- Place both feet flat on the floor.
- Sit tall.
- Relax your shoulders down.
- Place your right hand on the seat behind you and the other hand on the steering wheel.
- Inhale and begin to rotate to your right side, starting at the navel.
- Exhale and continue to work your way up the torso, twisting from the bottom of the ribs, chest, shoulders, and finally, head and neck.
- Keep your chin level and look back behind you as far as you can.
- Hold the twist for 5 to 10 breaths on each side.
- Gently unwind and repeat the opposite way.

Notice where it's easy to twist and where it's more difficult. Focus more on the areas that don't twist well

....

When twisting toward the door, grab hold of the handle or seatbelt to securely twist

....

Do not round or arch your back while twisting

....

Try this in the driver's seat, a chair, or the edge of your sleeper

....

Do this every time you buckle up and don't forget to move the opposite way

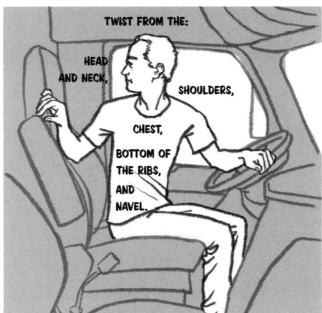

PELVIC TILTS

Long bouts of sitting can wreak havoc on your lower back. Pelvic tilting is an easy way to relieve tension, tightness, and increase circulation to the lower body. Plus, you can do it safely while driving.

- Sit tall and hold the steering wheel securely.
- Inhale and arch your back as far as you can away from the seat.
- Feel your tailbone try to turn back toward the seat behind you.
- Lift your chest and draw your shoulder blades together toward your spine.
- Exhale, cross your arms on the steering wheel, and round your body back toward the seat.
- Tuck your head in and tailbone under, making your body into a C position.
- Repeat these two movements 5 to 15 times in a row.

Hold each position longer if it feels good to do so

....

If you are driving and doing this movement, just work with the lower body to stay focused on the road

....

Try this movement sitting in the driver's seat, a chair, or on all fours on your sleeper or on the floor

....

Repeat this sequence 2 to 4 times daily

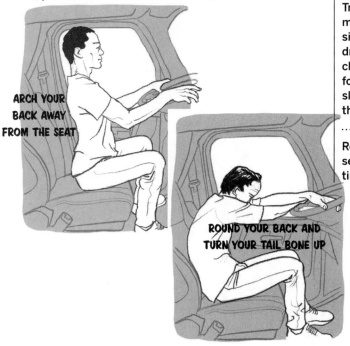

ARCH YOUR BACK AWAY FROM THE SEAT

ROUND YOUR BACK AND TURN YOUR TAIL BONE UP

UPPER BACK STRETCH

Improper sitting and one-handed driving or leaning can cause upper back, shoulder, and neck strain. Give your upper back a break with this quick stretch.

- Place both feet flat on the floor.
- Sit tall.
- Interlace your fingers together.
- Exhale and round your back like a C, allowing your tailbone to tuck under and your head to drop.
- Press your arms out in front of you and turn your palms to face away from you.
- Feel the stretch between your shoulder blades as you breathe.
- Hold this stretch for 5 to 10 breaths.

Move your arms up and down or side to side to change and enhance the stretch

....

Repeat 1 to 3 times daily

....

Do this stretch in your driver's seat, a chair, at the edge of your sleeper, or while standing

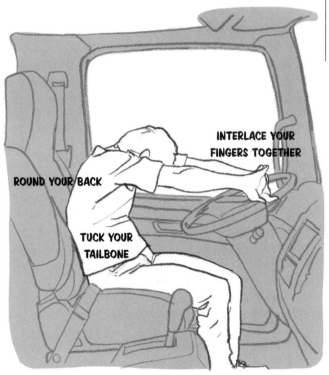

ROUND YOUR BACK

INTERLACE YOUR FINGERS TOGETHER

TUCK YOUR TAILBONE

CORE FLOAT

Decomplicate core work. This is a quick move you can insert into your day anytime you are sitting (and don't need your feet). The moment you lift your legs, you will feel your core muscles kick in. Instant core success!

- Find a seat.
- Lengthen your spine.
- Relax your shoulders down.
- Lean back slightly and lift your legs.
- Hold that floating position for 5 counts or 5 breaths.
- Repeat often!

Try this on a chair, bench, the driver's seat, or edge of your sleeper

....

Options: Lift only one leg or play with the height of your legs to change the core challenge

....

Hold onto the chair for more support or let go and move your arms out in front of you, above you, or out to a "T" to challenge your core

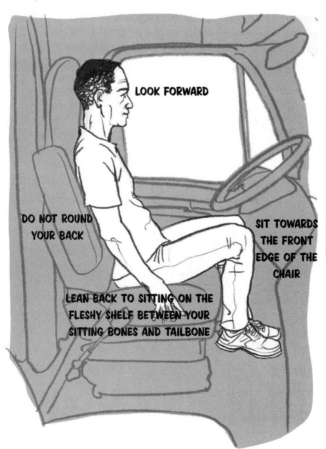

LOOK FORWARD

DO NOT ROUND YOUR BACK

SIT TOWARDS THE FRONT EDGE OF THE CHAIR

LEAN BACK TO SITTING ON THE FLESHY SHELF BETWEEN YOUR SITTING BONES AND TAILBONE

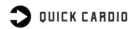

CHAIR RUNNING

Getting cardio in as a truck driver can be difficult. Get your heart rate up quickly, and all while you are sitting down. This move doubles as a great core strengthener and stabilizer, too.

- Sit down in the driver's seat, sleeper, or on a chair.
- Sit away from the backrest.
- Place your feet flat on the floor.
- Lengthen your spine.
- Relax your shoulders down.
- Grab hold of the chair on each side for more stability.
- Begin to slowly lift and lower your legs up off the ground.
- Only lift as high as you can keep your body from rounding.
- Gently touch one foot down and lift the opposite.
- After 30 seconds, begin to speed up the movement like you are starting to run.

Hold onto the chair or move your arms like you are running

....

Play with the pace of your run to create more of a cardio experience

....

Work to increase your chair running time from 1 minute up to 5 minutes

....

Move your arms as if you were running to get your heart rate up even more

....

Continue to chair run for 1 minute, repeat again 1 to 2 more times

....

Sequence: 30 second slow run -> 30 second run -> 30 second rest -> Repeat 2 more times

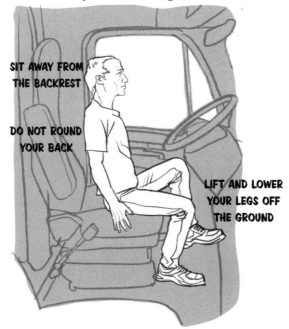

SIT AWAY FROM THE BACKREST

DO NOT ROUND YOUR BACK

LIFT AND LOWER YOUR LEGS OFF THE GROUND

6. SLEEPER, NOT JUST FOR SLEEPING

Your bed is made for more than just lying around and sleeping. And what's worse than sleeping in your bed is not sleeping in your bed. Use your bed as an opportunity to shut your body off and turn your body on for the day in a more caring way.

Many drivers find that when they lie down to go to bed, they try to fall asleep and wonder why they can't. Although there are dozens of reasons why that may be difficult, adding a few stretches before bed can help relax your body and assist you into a blissful sleep.

When you wake up, take a few minutes and move, stretch, breathe. Like taking a car out of storage, you have to lubricate the joints and get the fluids moving again before you run the car. The same is true for your body.

Where can you find time to get down on the ground and strike a pose? By looking at your bed, the ground, or any flat surface as an opportunity to lubricate your joints, breathe life into your body, or relax your muscles and mind. To get moving more, you will begin to see an increase in your ability to do what you love and love that you are able to do it.

SEATED CAT-COW

Reduce back, shoulder, and neck pain quickly with an easy move you can do right on your sleeper.

- Sit on the sleeper or floor with your legs crossed.
- Interlace your fingers and extend your arms up overhead and pull them back as far behind your ears as you can.
- Take a deep breath in and arch your back as much as you can.
- Exhale and round your back.
- If sitting with crossed legs is uncomfortable, try this seated at the edge of the sleeper, or on a chair.
- Repeat this movement 5 to 10 times in a row.

Options: Sit with legs out straight in front of you, knees bent, or on a chair

....

Exaggerate this movement as much as possible to bring your whole body into it

....

Do this movement 1 to 3 times a day

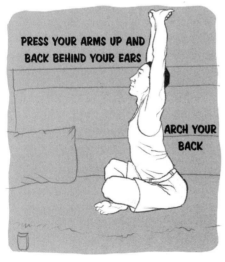

PRESS YOUR ARMS UP AND BACK BEHIND YOUR EARS

ARCH YOUR BACK

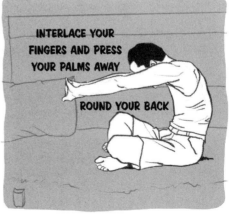

INTERLACE YOUR FINGERS AND PRESS YOUR PALMS AWAY

ROUND YOUR BACK

BOUND ANGLE

Improve circulation and stretch the groin, inner thighs, and hips, while helping to soothe sciatica.

- Start seated on the sleeper or floor.
- Bring the bottom of the feet together.
- Inhale and sit tall.
- Exhale and begin to fold forward from your hips.
- Extend through the chest and crown of your head.
- Hold this stretch for 10 breaths.

Do not round your back

....

If knee pain or hip pain is present, slide your feet further forward

....

Try holding your feet together or reaching your arms forward

....

Press down on your knees with your elbows to increase the hip stretch

....

Try this pose before you go to bed

....

Repeat 1 to 2 times daily

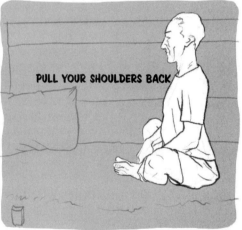

PULL YOUR SHOULDERS BACK

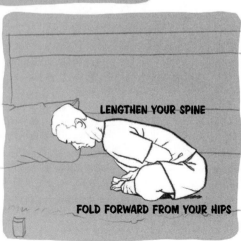

LENGTHEN YOUR SPINE

FOLD FORWARD FROM YOUR HIPS

STAR POSE

A quick outer hip and thigh stretch will help with knee, hip, and lower back pain.

- Start seated on the sleeper or floor.
- Bring the bottom of the feet together and slide them away from your hips to create a diamond shape.
- Inhale and sit tall.
- Exhale and begin to fold forward from your hips.
- Extend through the chest and crown of your head.
- Hold this stretch for 10 breaths.

If knee pain or hip pain is present, slide your feet further forward or support your knees with pillows

....

Try this pose before bed

....

Repeat 1 to 2 times daily

....

Pair this with Bond Angle for a complete hip release

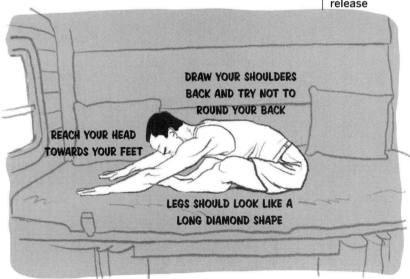

DRAW YOUR SHOULDERS BACK AND TRY NOT TO ROUND YOUR BACK

REACH YOUR HEAD TOWARDS YOUR FEET

LEGS SHOULD LOOK LIKE A LONG DIAMOND SHAPE

FIGURE FOUR (PIRIFORMIS STRETCH)

Unlock tight hips and release your sore back. This pose is helpful for reducing symptoms of sciatica and some forms of knee pain.

Seated version

- Start seated at the edge of your sleeper or chair.
- Sit tall and take a deep breath in.
- Cross your right ankle over the opposite knee and flex your foot.
- As you exhale, hinge at the hips and fold forward.
- Draw the shoulders back to keep the chest open.
- Hold this for 5 to 10 breaths.
- Repeat on the opposite side.

To increase the stretch, gently press down on the crossed leg with your right elbow

....

If you feel pinching in the knee or groin, grab the thigh and externally rotate it (outward) to make space

....

Extend the chest and head forward to create a deeper stretch in the back and hips

....

Repeat 1 to 4 times daily

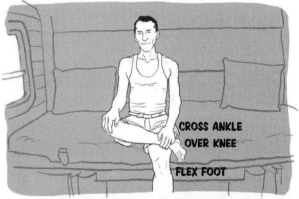

CROSS ANKLE
OVER KNEE

FLEX FOOT

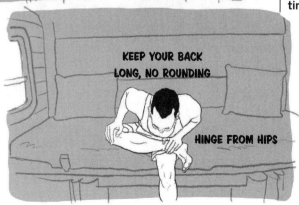

KEEP YOUR BACK
LONG, NO ROUNDING

HINGE FROM HIPS

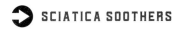
Lying Down Version

Try the lying down version if it is difficult to cross the ankle over the knee.

- Start by lying down.
- Cross one ankle over the opposite knee and flex your foot.
- If the head, neck, and torso are not in line, support your head with a pillow.
- **OPTION 1:** Press your crossed leg away from your body with or without the assistance of your hands.
- **OPTION 2:** Draw your legs in toward you and grab hold of the lower legs (shin and/or hamstring) or loop a belt underneath the hamstring and grab hold.
- Breathe calmly and lengthen the spine from head to tailbone.
- Press your back pants pockets down onto the bed as you draw your legs in.
- Hold this stretch for 5 to 10 breaths.
- Repeat on the opposite side.

Support your head with a pillow if your neck is not comfortable

....

Continue to press outward on the crossed leg with your elbow to increase the stretch

....

Use a strap, belt, or towel to hold the bottom leg if you can't grab hold

....

Repeat this stretch before you go to bed each night

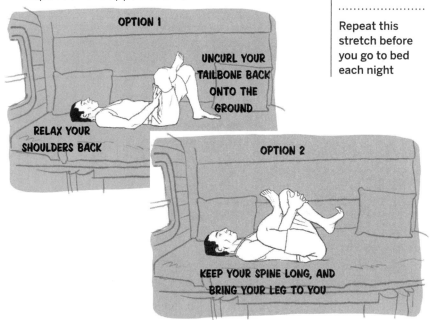

OPTION 1

UNCURL YOUR TAILBONE BACK ONTO THE GROUND

RELAX YOUR SHOULDERS BACK

OPTION 2

KEEP YOUR SPINE LONG, AND BRING YOUR LEG TO YOU

WINDSHIELD WIPERS HIP STRETCH

The older we get, the stiffer our hips become. Keeping hips mobile can help reduce back injuries and involves a great stretch after a long day.

- Lie down on the sleeper or the floor.
- Bend your knees and place your feet wider than your hips.
- Take a deep breath in, and as you exhale, drop your knees to the left.
- Turn your head to the right.
- Breathe calmly and deeply.
- Hold this stretch for 5 to 10 breaths or until tightness subsides.
- Repeat on the opposite side.
- Repeat this in the morning when you wake up and at night before you go to bed.

Allow the hip and lower back to arch on the inward knee side

....

Experiment holding the stretch or to change the stretch move back and forth in repetition like windshield wipers

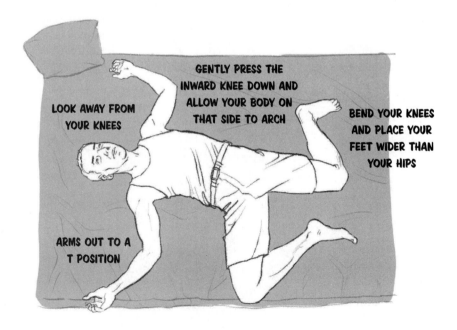

LOOK AWAY FROM YOUR KNEES

GENTLY PRESS THE INWARD KNEE DOWN AND ALLOW YOUR BODY ON THAT SIDE TO ARCH

BEND YOUR KNEES AND PLACE YOUR FEET WIDER THAN YOUR HIPS

ARMS OUT TO A T POSITION

BEGINNER'S BACK STRETCH SPHINX

To counterbalance the constant flexion of the body and continual driving position, the sphinx helps to stretch the hip flexors, abdomen, chest muscles, and lower back.

- Begin by lying down on your belly.
- Actively lengthen your legs out behind you.
- Slide your arms out in front of you at shoulder distance.
- Feel the chest widen and draw up on your belly as your tailbone sinks between your thighs.
- Stretch from the crown of your head to the tips of your toes.
- Hold this stretch for 5 to 10 breaths; repeat this 2 to 3 more times.
- Repeat 1 to 3 times daily as a great stretch before bed

Spread your fingers wide and press down through your hands

....

Stretch your legs long and press the tops of your feet into the bed

....

This stretch is a great alternative to Back Stretch Cobra

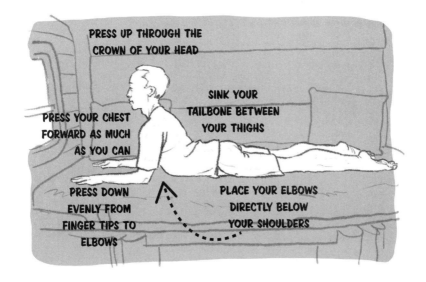

PRESS UP THROUGH THE CROWN OF YOUR HEAD

SINK YOUR TAILBONE BETWEEN YOUR THIGHS

PRESS YOUR CHEST FORWARD AS MUCH AS YOU CAN

PRESS DOWN EVENLY FROM FINGER TIPS TO ELBOWS

PLACE YOUR ELBOWS DIRECTLY BELOW YOUR SHOULDERS

BACK STRETCH COBRA

Another option when your back and hips are tight, stiff, and sore, and you are feeling the effects of long-term sitting.

- Begin by lying down on your belly.
- Actively lengthen your legs out behind you.
- Slide your hands to start underneath your shoulders with your elbows lifted off the bed.
- Take a deep breath in. and as you exhale, pull back on your hands, and begin to rise.
- Relax your shoulders and turn your elbows inward toward your body.
- Hold this stretch for 5 to 10 breaths, repeat this 2 to 3 more times.

Only come as high as you can while still feeling your back and core muscles doing the work

. . . .

Pull back on your hands instead of pushing up with your hands

. . . .

Pull back on your hands to help your chest move even further forward

. . . .

Repeat 1 to 3 times daily as a great stretch before bed

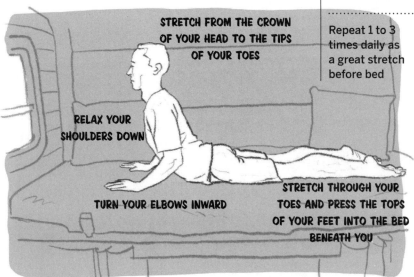

STRETCH FROM THE CROWN OF YOUR HEAD TO THE TIPS OF YOUR TOES

RELAX YOUR SHOULDERS DOWN

TURN YOUR ELBOWS INWARD

STRETCH THROUGH YOUR TOES AND PRESS THE TOPS OF YOUR FEET INTO THE BED BENEATH YOU

DEVOTIONAL BACK STRETCH

Life can be stressful. Find complete relaxation of your body and brain with this back stretch. Ahhhh. It's not just about physical relief. It's about mental relief, as well.

- Start on all fours on the sleeper or the floor.
- Exhale and sit your hips back.
- Stretch your arms as far forward as they can go and relax your shoulders down.
- Hold this for 5 to 10 breaths.

Support ankles with a rolled towel

....

Spread the knees wide to make room for the belly or chest

....

Support the head on a pillow or rolled towel

....

Your hips may not meet your heels, and that is okay

....

Breathe deeply and relax your hips back with each breath

....

Repeat before you go to bed each night

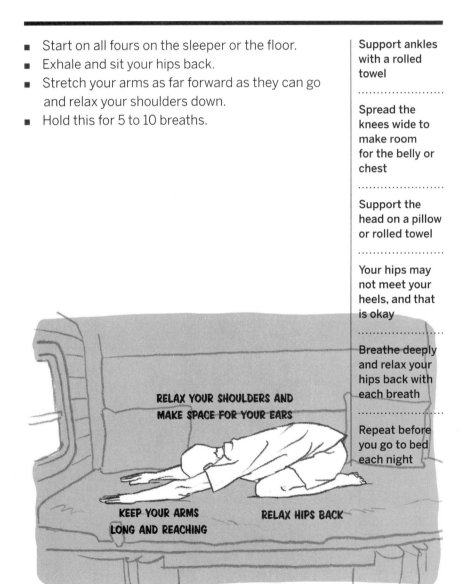

RELAX YOUR SHOULDERS AND MAKE SPACE FOR YOUR EARS

KEEP YOUR ARMS LONG AND REACHING

RELAX HIPS BACK

HEART OPENER

Strengthen your back as you soothe your shoulders and open your chest. This pose will help you counterbalance the effects of slouching and poor posture due to long-term sitting and driving.

- Start on your hands and knees on the sleeper or floor.
- Walk your hands forward of your shoulders and sit your hips up and back.
- Rest on the forehead and chin, and support your head if necessary with a pillow or rolled blanket.
- Drop your front ribs, and as you exhale, draw your belly in.
- Continue to breathe, and as you do, sink into your underarms.
- Hold this for 5 to 10 breaths.

Your knees should be at a place where you don't feel the need to sit back

....

Afterward, slide back to sit toward your heels

....

Repeat 1 to 2 times a day

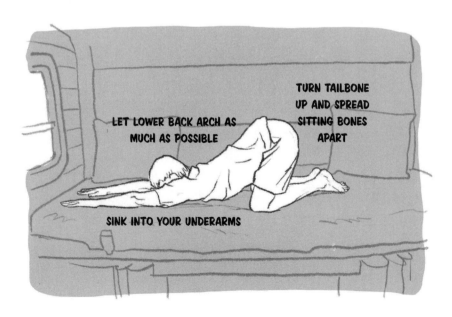

TURN TAILBONE UP AND SPREAD SITTING BONES APART

LET LOWER BACK ARCH AS MUCH AS POSSIBLE

SINK INTO YOUR UNDERARMS

SEATED SIDE BEND

Side bending is a simple way to stretch and tone the obliques, back, and abdominal muscles while improving flexibility in the spine. When you spend too much time sitting and even less time reaching, your body stiffens up. Let's do something about that.

- Begin seated on the edge of the sleeper or a chair.
- Place your feet flat on the floor.
- Inhale and lift one arm up overhead.
- Exhale and side bend your body to the opposite side.
- Breathe into the stretching side; imagine breaking the ribs apart with each inhale.
- Gaze in a direction that is comfortable for the head and neck.
- Hold this stretch for 5 to 10 breaths.
- Repeat on the opposite side.

Try rolling the torso open or slightly closed to change the line of stretch you feel

....

Hold the head with the top hand by bending at the elbow if needed

....

Repeat this side bend wherever you are just sitting around throughout the day (2 to 4 times daily)

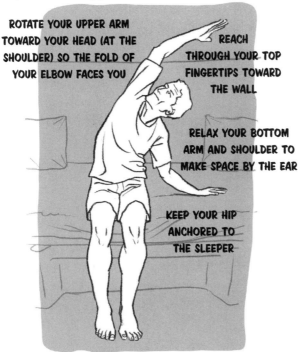

ROTATE YOUR UPPER ARM TOWARD YOUR HEAD (AT THE SHOULDER) SO THE FOLD OF YOUR ELBOW FACES YOU

REACH THROUGH YOUR TOP FINGERTIPS TOWARD THE WALL

RELAX YOUR BOTTOM ARM AND SHOULDER TO MAKE SPACE BY THE EAR

KEEP YOUR HIP ANCHORED TO THE SLEEPER

SEATED SPINAL TWIST

Twisting is a wonderful way to nourish the spine and give relief to the muscles of the back and abdomen. Breathe deeply here and create space within the muscles of the ribs (intercostal muscles).

- Start seated at the edge of your sleeper or a chair.
- Plant your feet flat on the floor.
- Place your left hand on your right knee and your right hand behind your back.
- Take a deep breath in, and as you exhale, allow your body to rotate.
- Inhale, and as you exhale, work your way up through your body from bottom to top.
- First, rotate from your navel.
- Second, rotate from your rib cage and heart.
- Finally, rotate your head, neck, and eyes.
- Hold this stretch for 5 breaths and slowly return back to center.
- Repeat on the opposite side.
- Look for other times throughout the day you can add in this twist.

Keep your hips level and anchored and do not twist your pelvis

....

Do this twist each time you have to buckle up, and don't forget the opposite side

....

Notice which side is tighter and hold that position for a few extra breaths

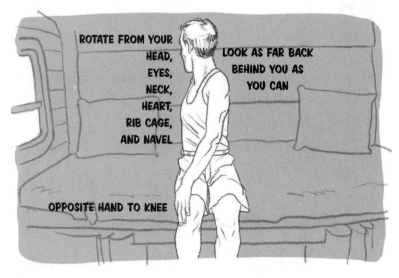

ROTATE FROM YOUR HEAD, EYES, NECK, HEART, RIB CAGE, AND NAVEL

LOOK AS FAR BACK BEHIND YOU AS YOU CAN

OPPOSITE HAND TO KNEE

FULL-BODY STRETCH

Full-body stretch is a simple way to break free from the tension, tightness, and restriction our bodies feel when we just don't move enough. Unlock your body and your breath with this supine stretch.

- Lie down on your sleeper or the floor.
- Remove any pillows from underneath you.
- Inhale and stretch your arms up overhead.
- Exaggerate the movement as much as possible.
- Exhale and let your belly completely deflate.
- Continue to breathe deeply and stretch from fingertips to toes.
- Hold this for 5 to 10 breaths.
- Repeat this in the morning when you wake up and in the evening before you go to bed.

Try adding in a side bend by moving your upper and lower body to one side, grabbing one wrist and pulling, or crossing your ankles and squeezing

....

Play around with the stretch by adding in a little side bend or reaching through one leg or arm more than the other

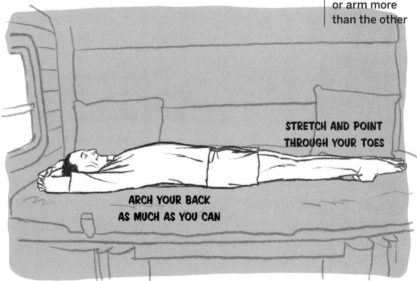

STRETCH AND POINT THROUGH YOUR TOES

ARCH YOUR BACK AS MUCH AS YOU CAN

FULL BODY RELAXATION

Creating time to lie down with your eyes closed and body still is necessary for the body to relax and restore itself. Taking an adult time-out like this can help reduce blood pressure and calm your nervous system.

- Lie down on your back on the sleeper or the floor.
- Place one hand on your belly and one hand on your chest.
- Slide the legs a little wider than hip distance or until they can relax.
- Soften your shoulders and begin to pay attention to your breathing.
- Follow your inhale by breathing into the lower hand and feeling your belly rise, and then your chest expand.
- Exhale and feel the chest relax down and the belly release all the air out.
- Repeat this cycle of inhaling for 4 counts and exhaling for 8 counts.

Support the head if the upper back and neck are tight

....

Breathe slowly and steadily for 5 to 10 minutes

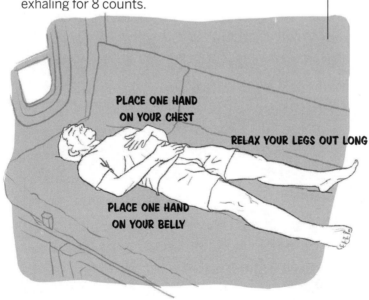

PLACE ONE HAND ON YOUR CHEST

RELAX YOUR LEGS OUT LONG

PLACE ONE HAND ON YOUR BELLY

RECLINED BOUND ANGLE LOWER BACK RELAXATION

Pairing a hip stretch with the breathing relaxation sequence can help both your body and mind relax at the end of a long day.

- Following the same directions as above, relax your entire body.
- Place the bottoms of the feet together and slide them out away from you to a place where your hips are relaxed and your body is at ease.
- You may choose to support the knees with pillows.
- Turn your palms to face up and focus on your breathing.
- Slowly and calmly inhale for 4 counts and exhale for 8 counts.
- Repeat this breathing relaxation sequence for 5 to 10 minutes to prepare for bed or as a mini relaxation session during the day.

Practice these relaxation techniques before you go to bed or when you need to rest your body in place of a nap

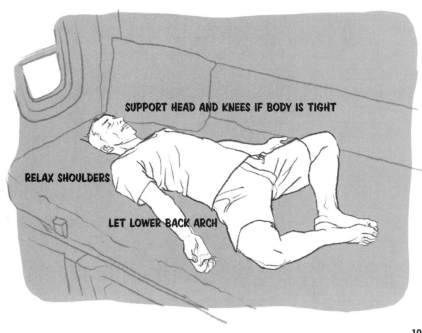

SUPPORT HEAD AND KNEES IF BODY IS TIGHT

RELAX SHOULDERS

LET LOWER BACK ARCH

STRAP STRETCH SERIES

While each of the following stretches can be performed individually, **The Sleeper Leg and Hip Strap Stretch Series** *can also be done as a sequence. Complete all of the stretches in this series on one side of your body, then repeat the series on the opposite side of your body.*

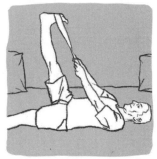
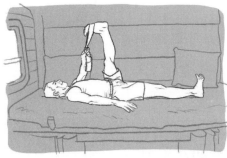

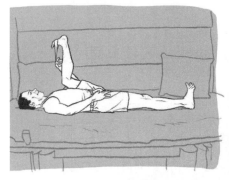
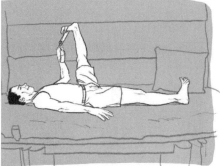

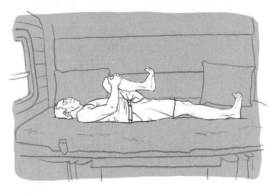

SLEEPER RECLINED HAMSTRING STRETCH

Long-term sitting can shorten and tighten the backs of the legs, leaving it difficult to walk and sleep. Stretching the hamstrings can help you increase mobility and allow you to function optimally throughout the day, while reducing other symptoms like foot pain, back pain, and neck pain.

- Lie down on your back on the sleeper or the floor.
- Loop strap (belt or towel) over the ball of one foot and extend the leg out to 45 degrees.
- Keep your pelvis steady and stable.
- Hold the strap with your arm at full extension.
- Hold for 5 to 10 breaths.

Keep your bottom leg bent or straight

....

Slowly draw your leg in toward you little by little only as the stretch fades

....

Keep your arms fully extended with shoulders relaxed

....

Only draw your leg in until you feel a gentle stretch

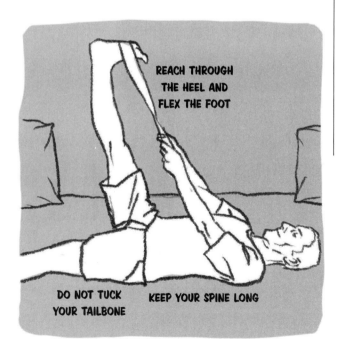

REACH THROUGH THE HEEL AND FLEX THE FOOT

DO NOT TUCK YOUR TAILBONE   KEEP YOUR SPINE LONG

SLEEPER OUTER HIP AND LEG STRETCH

A long day of sitting can create tightness in the inner thighs. The inner thighs are like a drawstring bag for the lower back: loosening them may help reduce back pain. Regularly stretching the inner thigh and groin can improve range of motion, flexibility, and circulation.

- Hold the strap with the opposite hand as your strapped leg.
- Slowly cross your leg over the midline of the body a few inches.
- Press the outer hip of the lifted leg down into the ground.
- Hold for 5 to 10 breaths.

Move the upper leg around to change the stretch

....

Avoid rolling your ankle, keep it straight

....

Bend your knee slightly if necessary

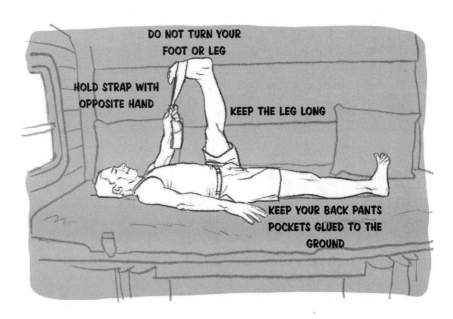

DO NOT TURN YOUR FOOT OR LEG

HOLD STRAP WITH OPPOSITE HAND

KEEP THE LEG LONG

KEEP YOUR BACK PANTS POCKETS GLUED TO THE GROUND

SLEEPER INNER THIGH AND GROIN STRETCH

Inner thigh restriction can cause lower back pain. Open up your hips to help create an increased range of motion throughout the day. Stretching the outer hip and thigh may help reduce knee and hip pain when done regularly.

- Bring the leg back to the center.
- Take the strap with the same hand as your leg.
- Keep your hips steady and your core toned (like someone is going to step on your belly).
- With foot flexed, extend the leg out away from your body.
- Hold for 5 to 10 breaths.

Engage your core to help keep the hips down

....

Hold at a point where you can feel a stretch in your inner thigh

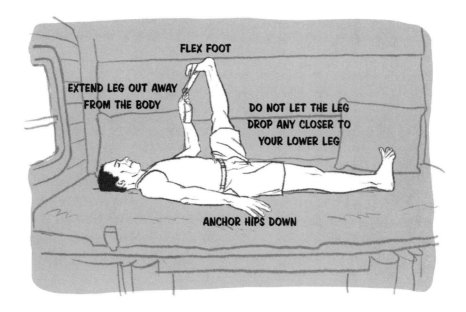

FLEX FOOT

EXTEND LEG OUT AWAY FROM THE BODY

DO NOT LET THE LEG DROP ANY CLOSER TO YOUR LOWER LEG

ANCHOR HIPS DOWN

SLEEPER HAPPY BABY HIP STRETCH

Use this move to stretch the hip flexors (of the straight leg), hamstrings, and groin. The perfect stretch after a long day. Practicing this stretch regularly will help you increase flexibility and mobility, allowing your body to move more freely and with less pain and discomfort.

- Bring the leg back to the center.
- Pull down on the strap to bend your knee.
- Draw your heel to sit above your knee.
- Press your knee toward the ground.
- Hold for 5 to 10 breaths.

The goal is not to touch the ground, but rather feel a stretch in the outer hip and thigh

....

Do not lift your hips

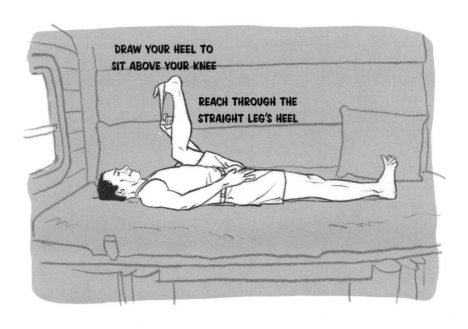

DRAW YOUR HEEL TO SIT ABOVE YOUR KNEE

REACH THROUGH THE STRAIGHT LEG'S HEEL

SLEEPER KNEE HUG

Breathe and relax with a hug of the leg. This pose is great after a long day when your body is struggling to let go. Hugging the knee into the chest releases the hip and hamstring and increases your range of motion, while the straight leg is focused on opening the hip after a long day of sitting.

- Release the strap and pull your knee into your chest.
- Hold for 5 to 10 breaths.
- Release the leg and rest for several breaths.
- Repeat on the opposite side.

Slide the bent knee to the side if you need more space around your middle

....

Loop the strap over your shin to better grab hold of the leg

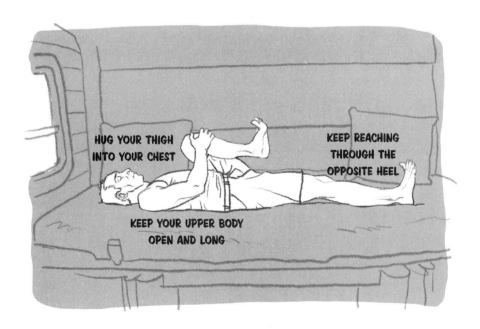

HUG YOUR THIGH INTO YOUR CHEST

KEEP REACHING THROUGH THE OPPOSITE HEEL

KEEP YOUR UPPER BODY OPEN AND LONG

7. OUTSIDE YOUR RIG

The world is your playground, and it is up to you to play on it. Getting up and moving around isn't always possible as a truck driver, but during those moments you can, I want to encourage you to double-down and get the most bang for your buck. That means you strike a pose. Get up and move, breathe, and enjoy life.

The best way to do that is to move about. Every time you are outside the truck, ask yourself what you could be doing right now. Look around you and see what is available. Your truck step, your tire, a bench, inside your trailer? Use that space. What do you have lying around? Water jug? Bag of tools? Step ladder? Pretend those are weights. Take a lap around your truck for a quick inspection. Those are steps you wouldn't have otherwise taken.

When you catch yourself sitting and waiting for the dock to open or for your pickup time to arrive, get up and get out of your truck and move. Bend forward, bend backward, twist, squat, reach. Each of those movements is an opportunity for your body to stretch, your heart rate to rise, and your blood to pump. You have an opportunity to break the mold in your mind for how you think movement should be experienced, for how life is supposed to be lived.

Who says you can't do yoga in a parking lot? Who says you would look silly stretching on your truck step? What if those moves inspire another driver to start moving again? What if your decision to do that side bend to get rid of that pesky back pain shows another trucker it's okay to do that, too? And the real movement becomes more truck drivers just like you living a more active life.

FUNCTIONAL CALF STRETCH (PLANTAR FASCIITIS)

Calf tightness can cause foot pain and knee pain and problems when walking, as well as restrict blood flow back to the heart, as the calf is the hydraulic pump (second heart) for the lower body's blood flow. When restricted by tightness, these functions are limited.

- Standing tall, casually step back with one foot.
- Turn both feet to point forward and check the back foot's heel to make sure it's not turned in.
- Square your hips forward.
- Inhale and bend your front knee to rest over your ankle.
- Exhale and bend your back knee as much as you can without lifting the heel.
- Slowly bend and straighten the back knee 10 times.
- Repeat this on the opposite side.

You do not need a large stride (smaller is better)

....

Keep your feet hip distance or wider (think two water skis)

....

Keep the back knee moving in line with the toes

....

Repeat this regularly throughout the day 2 to 4 times

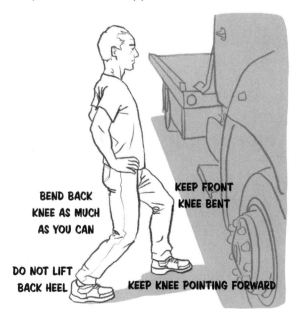

BEND BACK KNEE AS MUCH AS YOU CAN

KEEP FRONT KNEE BENT

DO NOT LIFT BACK HEEL

KEEP KNEE POINTING FORWARD

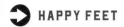

TIRE CALF STRETCH (FOR PLANTAR FASCIITIS)

Release the calf muscle, Achilles tendon, and plantar tendon (calf, ankle, and foot) from tension and restriction. Great for plantar fasciitis (pain in the bottom of the foot) and foot problems.

- Stand tall facing your truck tire or a wall.
- Step one foot up and place the ball of the foot against the tire or a wall.
- Square the hips forward.
- Gently lean into the truck, stretching the back of the front leg.
- Hold this stretch for 5 to 10 breaths or until the stretch fades.
- Repeat on the opposite side.
- Practice this stretch 1 to 4 times daily.

Do this stretch several times throughout the day

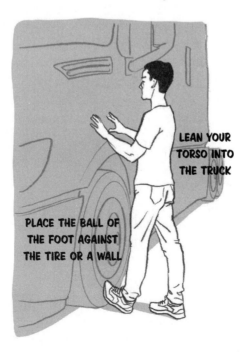

LEAN YOUR TORSO INTO THE TRUCK

PLACE THE BALL OF THE FOOT AGAINST THE TIRE OR A WALL

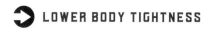

TRUCK STEP SERIES

While each of the following stretches can be performed individually,
The Truck Step Series *can also be done as a mini-sequence. This mini-sequence is a total body flow involving toning and stretching of the legs and hips. You will also activate your obliques as you stretch your back and spine and relieve tension in the neck. Practice this mini-sequence once a day.*

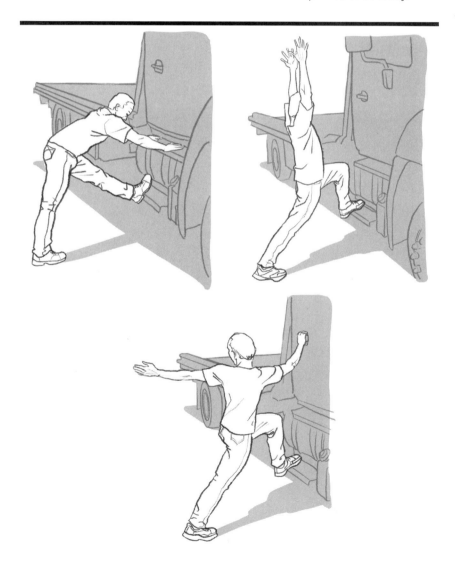

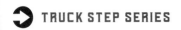
TRUCK STEP ONE-LEGGED HAMSTRING STRETCH

- Begin by facing your truck and step one foot up onto the lower step.
- Reach down and place your hands on the top step.
- Slowly begin to lengthen the front leg.
- Exhale and slowly fold toward the leg.
- Hold this pose for 5 to 10 breaths.

To increase the stretch use your hand to draw the front leg's hip back

....

Do not lock the front leg's knee

....

Bend the back knee to help you hinge further forward

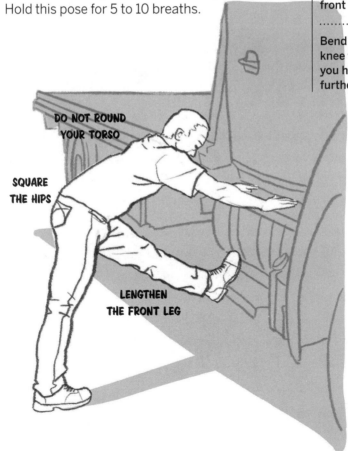

DO NOT ROUND YOUR TORSO

SQUARE THE HIPS

LENGTHEN THE FRONT LEG

TRUCK STEP LUNGE

The truck step is the perfect place to get a little movement in. Use this pose to counterbalance long bouts of sitting, helping you increase circulation to the lower body, reduce back pain, and improve mobility in the upper body by reducing restriction in the legs.

- Rise up slowly from the Hamstring Stretch and bend your front knee.
- Keep the back foot facing forward and allow the heel to slightly rise.
- Inhale and lift your arms up overhead.
- Press into the front leg and feel the hamstring and glute activate.
- Hold this pose for 5 to 10 breaths.

Place your hands on the truck for more stability

....

Bend your back knee if your hips are tight

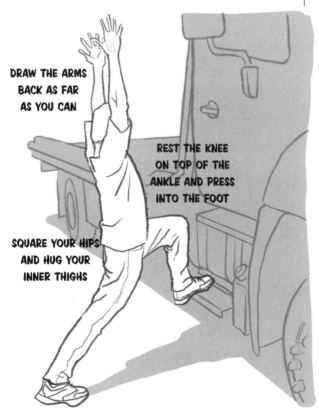

DRAW THE ARMS BACK AS FAR AS YOU CAN

REST THE KNEE ON TOP OF THE ANKLE AND PRESS INTO THE FOOT

SQUARE YOUR HIPS AND HUG YOUR INNER THIGHS

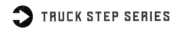

TRUCK STEP LUNGE AND TWIST

Twisting is an essential movement we all must do to age healthily. Add this stretch each time you get ready to step into your truck.

- Keep your front knee bent on the truck step.
- Drop your arms open to a T position.
- Slowly begin to rotate the body toward the front leg.
- As you twist, work from the bottom of the spine and work your way up.
- Hold this pose for 5 to 10 breaths.
- Repeat on the opposite side.

If needed, hold onto the truck with your front hand

....

Slowly come out of the pose and try a Half Down Dog (explained shortly)

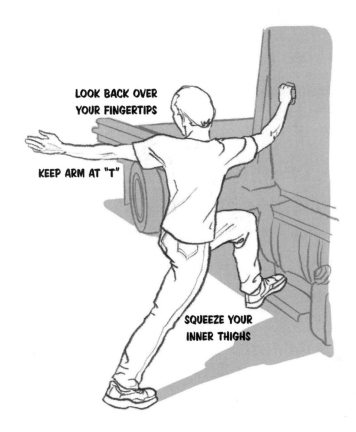

LOOK BACK OVER YOUR FINGERTIPS

KEEP ARM AT "T"

SQUEEZE YOUR INNER THIGHS

OBLIQUE SIDE STRETCH LUNGE

This lunging side bend stretches from foot to fingertips, focusing on the side body, especially the hips, obliques, and underarms.

- Stand with your shoulder next to the truck.
- Step back about a leg length with your outside foot.
- Balance on the ball of the back foot as you press back into your heel.
- Bend the front knee over the front ankle.
- Inhale and reach the outside arm and roll the arm in toward your head.
- Exhale and begin to side bend toward your truck.
- Hold the stretch for 1 to 5 breaths.
- Inhale slowly and come back up.
- Repeat this stretch on each side 1 to 10 times.

Try this by a wall or chair

....

Keep the top arm from rolling in front of your face

....

Drop back with your knee down

....

Practice this 1 to 2 times daily

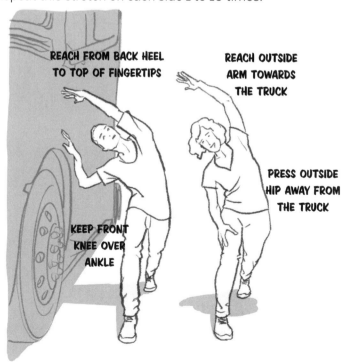

REACH FROM BACK HEEL TO TOP OF FINGERTIPS

REACH OUTSIDE ARM TOWARDS THE TRUCK

PRESS OUTSIDE HIP AWAY FROM THE TRUCK

KEEP FRONT KNEE OVER ANKLE

HALF DOWN DOG

Strike this pose whenever you are feeling stiff and tight (from heel to hip to hand) for a full back body stretch.

- Place your hands on the truck or a wall slightly higher than shoulder height.
- Take a big step back.
- As you exhale, begin to sink your head and chest down toward the ground.
- Breathe slowly and deeply for 5 to 10 breaths.
- Slowly bring your body back up to center.

Practice this against your truck, a wall, countertop, or chair

....

Continue to press into your hands and do not bend your elbows

....

Repeat this 1 to 4 times daily

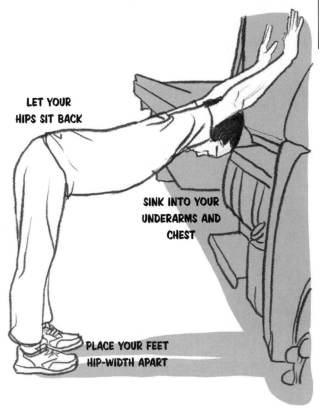

LET YOUR
HIPS SIT BACK

SINK INTO YOUR
UNDERARMS AND
CHEST

PLACE YOUR FEET
HIP-WIDTH APART

HANGING AROUND FULL-BODY RELEASE

Hanging decompresses the spine and can help to reduce pain and tightness. Look for all the places you can hang around during the day for a quick whole body release.

- Find a secure place above shoulder height to grab onto.
- Take a deep breath out and begin to relax your body downward.
- Bend your knees.
- Continue to deeply exhale and make your body feel heavy.
- Hold this hanging position for 5 to 10 breaths or as long as it feels good.

If you wish, take all the weight off your feet and hang on tight

....

Repeat this 1 to 3 times a day to help restore your body's mobility

....

You can hang just about anywhere: the side of your truck, pole, kitchen sink edge, monkey bar, or your truck step

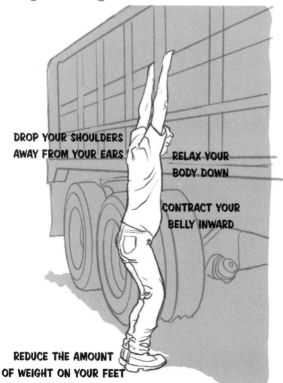

DROP YOUR SHOULDERS AWAY FROM YOUR EARS

RELAX YOUR BODY DOWN

CONTRACT YOUR BELLY INWARD

REDUCE THE AMOUNT OF WEIGHT ON YOUR FEET

HANGING AROUND HEEL, FOOT, AND CALF STRETCH

Within minutes of sitting, our calf muscles begin to shorten. Get a quick release every time you get back into the truck. Here's how:

- Step up onto the lower step of your truck.
- Securely grab hold somewhere on your truck.
- Keep your body tall.
- Sink one heel down off the step and hold for 3 to 5 breaths.
- Switch and repeat on the opposite side.
- Now drop both heels off the step and hold for 3 to 5 breaths.

You can also try this on the curb or your steps at home

....

Repeat this sequence 1 to 3 times a day or whenever you get back into the truck

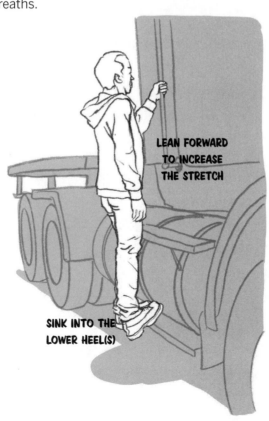

LEAN FORWARD TO INCREASE THE STRETCH

SINK INTO THE LOWER HEEL(S)

HANGING AROUND BACK & SHOULDER STRETCH

Improve shoulder health and mobility and release the lower back, sacrum, and tailbone.

- Start standing facing your truck door.
- Grab hold of the top step or somewhere on your truck securely.
- Take a deep breath in, and as you exhale, lean your hips back as far as you can.
- Soften in your shoulders and draw your belly in on the exhale.
- Hold this stretch for 5 to 10 breaths.

Try hanging and squatting, twisting and turning too

....

Find anything secure to grab onto and stretch

....

Relax your body but not your grip

....

Repeat 1 to 3 times daily

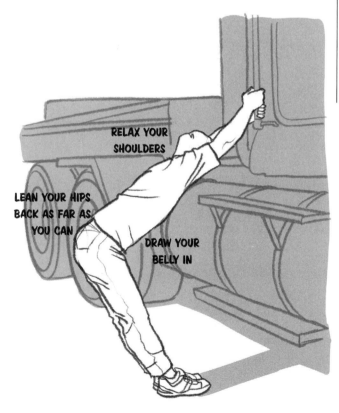

RELAX YOUR SHOULDERS

LEAN YOUR HIPS BACK AS FAR AS YOU CAN

DRAW YOUR BELLY IN

HANGING AROUND SIDE STRETCH

Use this stretch to eliminate that pesky lower back, hip, and shoulder pain, or restriction created from too much sitting or lack of mobility.

- Stand with your shoulder next to your truck.
- Grab onto the step—or some other secure spot no higher than shoulder height—with your inside arm.
- Step your inside foot to cross in front of your outside leg.
- Take a deep breath in, and as you exhale, lean into your side body, moving away from the truck.
- Reach your top arm up overhead and rotate the arm inward toward you.
- Breathe calmly and deeply for 5 to 10 breaths.
- Repeat on the opposite side.

Move your top arm, shoulders, or torso to change the stretch

....

Grab hold of anything nearby if not your truck step

....

Practice this stretch 1 to 2 times daily

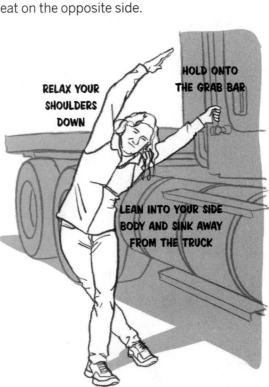

RELAX YOUR SHOULDERS DOWN

HOLD ONTO THE GRAB BAR

LEAN INTO YOUR SIDE BODY AND SINK AWAY FROM THE TRUCK

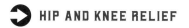

PANTS POCKET QUAD STRETCH

Stretch the knees, quadriceps, hip flexors, and abdomen all while challenging balance and stability. This quick move will improve posture and reduce strain from activities like running and sitting (I know, complete opposites).

- Start by standing next to your truck or another support.
- Bend one knee and tuck it behind you.
- Grab hold of the ankle and relax that shoulder down and back.
- Slowly begin to draw the heel toward your backside.
- Hold for 5 to 10 breaths.
- Slowly release down and repeat on the opposite side.

Lean up against the truck to help support your foot. Use your free hand to support you on your truck. If you are unable to connect the hand to the foot, loop a strap around the ankle of the bent leg

....

Keep your hips level

....

Practice this 1 to 2 times a day

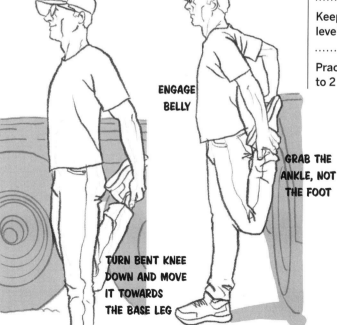

ENGAGE BELLY

GRAB THE ANKLE, NOT THE FOOT

TURN BENT KNEE DOWN AND MOVE IT TOWARDS THE BASE LEG

TRUCK PLANK

Tone your entire body and build up better core strength.

- Start on all fours.
- Without moving your upper body, step back with one foot at a time.
- Lean into your fingertips and press your body away from the floor.
- Hold this pose for 5 to 10 breaths.

If your wrists are sensitive, use a rolled towel under them

....

Challenge yourself and practice this daily, working up to a 1-minute hold or more

....

Practice this pose on your knees, forearms, or on the truck step for an Angled Truck Plank

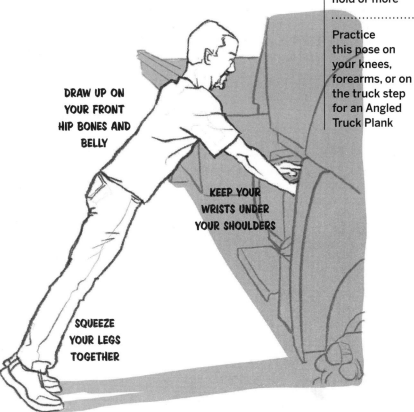

DRAW UP ON YOUR FRONT HIP BONES AND BELLY

KEEP YOUR WRISTS UNDER YOUR SHOULDERS

SQUEEZE YOUR LEGS TOGETHER

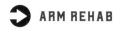

TRICEPS ANGLED PUSH-UP

Strengthen your upper back, triceps, and core with this truck-style push-up. Building up strength here will help improve posture and offer you a more toned upper body physique.

- Follow the setup for the truck plank.
- Place your hands on the upper step of your truck and take a big step back.
- Step your feet together.
- Tip your front hip bones up in toward your back.
- Turn the folds of your elbows to face the truck.
- Drop your shoulders and broaden your chest.
- Inhale slowly and lower your body only as far as you are able to stay in one long line.
- Exhale, squeeze your thighs, press your belly into your back body, and move back up into a plank position.
- Hold this pose for 5 to 10 breaths.

Try this on the ground or on your knees

....

Repeat this (3 to 10 times) only until you can no longer keep good form

....

Practice this 1 to 2 times daily

....

Move your body into Half Down Dog for a great counterpose

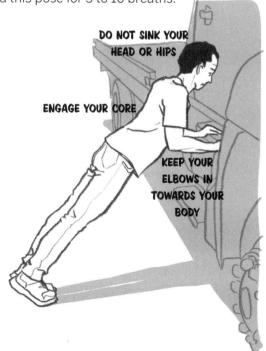

DO NOT SINK YOUR HEAD OR HIPS

ENGAGE YOUR CORE

KEEP YOUR ELBOWS IN TOWARDS YOUR BODY

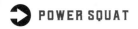

SQUAT IT DOWN (FUNCTIONAL SQUAT)

Squatting is an essential movement that stretches the legs, hips, and back. The more you squat, the easier it gets. When you have to bend down, try squatting down instead.

- Step your feet hip-width apart.
- Exhale, sit back into your hips and heels.
- Hold your weight (optional) at your chest.
- Inhale and rise up to standing by engaging your glutes and legs.
- Press the weight overhead.
- Add repetition and various speeds into the squat to make it more of a cardio exercise (3 count down, 1 count up / 2 count down, 2 count up / 1 count down, 3 count up / 1 count down, 1 count up).
- Change out the weight you hold in your hands, find things of various weight to change the load you carry, and change how hard your muscles work
- Repeat 10 times.

Can't sit back? Practice Functional Calf Release

....

Weight Options: water jug, hand weight, duffel bag, heavy hand tool

....

Play with the distance of your feet to change the squat muscle engagement

....

Repeat this 3 times a day

....

Move more quickly to create more of a cardio affect

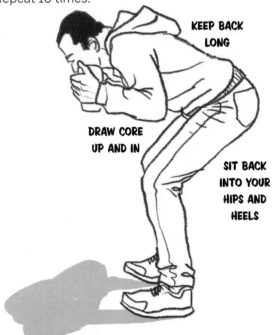

KEEP BACK LONG

DRAW CORE UP AND IN

SIT BACK INTO YOUR HIPS AND HEELS

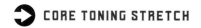

FUNCTIONAL STANDING CORE EXTENSION

10x your core! Stop training your core in flexion on the ground. Stand up! Stretch your hip flexors, lower back, and work your core muscles 10x better than a sit-up.

- Begin standing with your feet hip-width apart.
- Take a deep breath in.
- Inhale, bend your knees, and reach your arms up overhead.
- Drive your hips forward and reach your arms back.
- Exhale, return back to standing.
- Repeat this 10 times in a row.

Adjust the width of your feet to change the move

....

Add a weight in your hands

....

Do this when you get out of the truck (1 to 4 times a day)

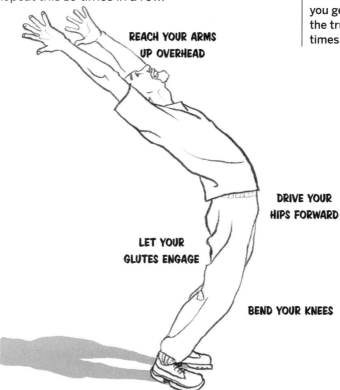

REACH YOUR ARMS UP OVERHEAD

DRIVE YOUR HIPS FORWARD

LET YOUR GLUTES ENGAGE

BEND YOUR KNEES

CARDIO STEP UP

Cardiovascular exercise is essential to our (heart) health. Cardio exercise isn't just running, biking or swimming. You can raise your heart rate right next to your truck as easy as stepping into your rig.

- Start standing facing your truck steps
- Take a deep breath in and a deep breath out.
- Inhale, step up onto the lower step of the truck.
- Immediately bring your opposite foot up to follow.
- Exhale step down one foot at a time.
- Repeat at a consistent pace for 1 minute.

Keep your body upright

....

Try not to lean forward

....

Hold onto the grab bar on your truck (if you have one) for more stability

....

Pick up the pace to increase your heart rate

....

Start out at 1 minute and work your way up to 5 minutes

EXTEND THROUGH THE TOP OF THE HEAD

MOVE YOUR ARMS IN COORDINATION WITH EACH STEP

KEEP YOUR BODY UPRIGHT

ENGAGE THE LOWER LEGS AND GLUTES WHEN STEPPING UP

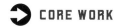
WATER JUG CORE

Never do a sit-up again. Use what you have and get a great core, back, and arm workout no matter where you are. Your core is 360 degrees around you. Don't forget your back muscles too.

- Start seated with your knees bent.
- Sit tall to begin.
- Rest the water jug on your chest and hold with hands.
- Relax your shoulders down.
- Exhale, gently tuck your tailbone. and slightly round your lower back.
- Inhale, lean back to 45 degrees.
- Exhale, rise back up to where you started.
- Inhale, press the water jug directly overhead.
- Exhale, place the water jug on your chest.
- Inhale, move back to a 45-degree angle.
- Repeat this cycle 5 to 10 times, for 1 to 3 cycles.

Focus on breathing into your side lungs and ribs

....

try adding a 7- to 9-inch mini ball behind you

....

For more of a challenge, extend your legs straight

....

Place something between your knees and squeeze for more core engagement

....

To adjust the weight, drink the water

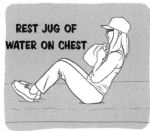

REST JUG OF WATER ON CHEST

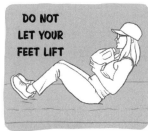

DO NOT LET YOUR FEET LIFT

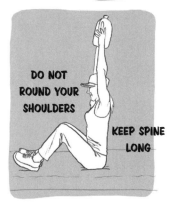

DO NOT ROUND YOUR SHOULDERS

KEEP SPINE LONG

WATER JUG SQUAT AND LIFT

Squats are a great way to tone the body and also get a bit of a cardio effect. Tone your legs, back, core and arms as you increase your heart rate, who said you need a gym to workout.

- Start by standing tall with your feet 3 to 4 feet apart.
- Turn your toes slightly out and press into the balls of the feet.
- Standing tall, relax your arms down in front of you holding the water jug in front of your hips.
- Inhale, press your legs straight and lift the water jug up over your head.
- Exhale, bend your knees, and lower the water jug down in front of you.
- Repeat this movement 10 to 20 times in a row.

Omit water jug and just lift your arms

....

Use another object or a weight to supplement the water jug

....

Drink water to reduce the weight of the jug

....

Try lifting your heels when you press your legs straight for an extra calf workout

....

For more of a calorie burn, add a pulse (slight bounce) at the bottom of the squat 3 to 10 times before you rise

....

Repeat your set of 10 to 20 2 or 3 more times for a more intense workout

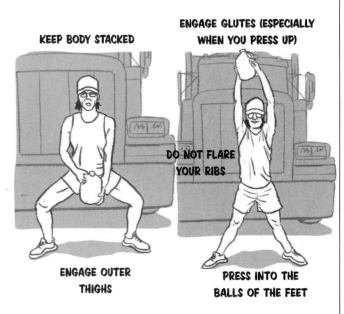

KEEP BODY STACKED

ENGAGE GLUTES (ESPECIALLY WHEN YOU PRESS UP)

DO NOT FLARE YOUR RIBS

ENGAGE OUTER THIGHS

PRESS INTO THE BALLS OF THE FEET

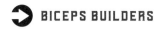
WATER JUG BICEPS CURL

Our modern lives require less and less of our upper body and that can mean muscle loss, so it is essential that we find more ways to build arm strength. Bicep curls are a great way to tone the arms and get you ready when it comes time to do some heavy lifting.

- Start out with your feet hips-width apart and your toes pointing forward.
- Grab hold of the water jug with your right hand and stand tall.
- Hinge from your hips and tip your torso 45-degrees forward.
- Keep your spine long and chin tucked in.
- Inhale and extend your water jug arm back and lift the jug up above your hip line.
- Exhale and curl your arm in towards your shoulder.
- Repeat this 10 to 15 times.
- Slowly come back up and repeat on the opposite side.

Drink water to reduce the weight of the jug

....

Do not allow your body to curl or lean when lifting the jug

....

Adjust the amount of repetitions to increase or decrease the challenge

....

Use a hand weight or something with weight if you do not have a water jug

....

Try doing both arms at the same time

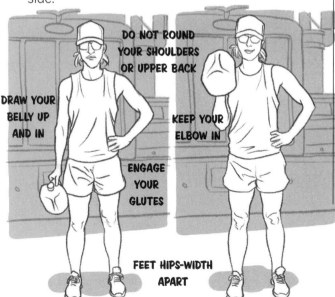

DO NOT ROUND YOUR SHOULDERS OR UPPER BACK

DRAW YOUR BELLY UP AND IN

KEEP YOUR ELBOW IN

ENGAGE YOUR GLUTES

FEET HIPS-WIDTH APART

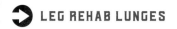
WATER JUG WALKING LUNGE

Add your water jug to your lunge for a great weight-bearing activity.

- Start standing with the jug at your chest.
- Inhale, step forward and lunge, keeping your body upright and tall.
- Exhale and step up to starting position.
- Continue to walk and lunge.
- Repeat this lunge 5 to 10 times on each side, 1 to 3 sets.

As you lunge, add a bicep curl, overhead press, or forward chest press with the jug

....

Try the Stationary Lunge: step forward into the lunge and step backward to center

....

Adjust the weight by drinking the water

....

Use a hand-weight or another prop if you do not have a water jug

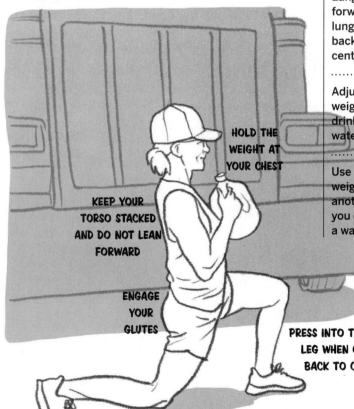

HOLD THE WEIGHT AT YOUR CHEST

KEEP YOUR TORSO STACKED AND DO NOT LEAN FORWARD

ENGAGE YOUR GLUTES

PRESS INTO THE FRONT LEG WHEN COMING BACK TO CENTER

FOOTWORK

Our feet are the foundation of our body and are made up of muscles, bones, and tissues, just like any other body part. And our feet spend too much time in shoes, leaving them immobile for much of the day. Take care of your feet to improve your body's health.

Toe Piano

- Take off your shoes and socks.
- Look at your feet on the floor.
- Spread your toes apart.
- Next, try to move your big toe without help and see if you can move your other toes.
- Repeat on the opposite foot.

Try rolling out the bottoms of the feet with a ball to help stimulate them

....

Use your hands to help separate your toes

....

And try to spread your toes on their own

....

Practice a minimum of 1 to 2 times a day

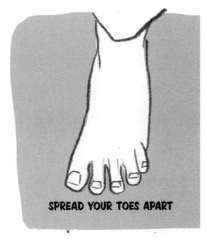

SPREAD YOUR TOES APART

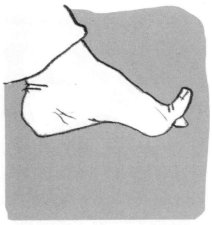

Dancer Feet

- Take off your shoes and socks.
- Spread your toes apart.
- Roll forward over the tops of your toes as far as your foot will allow.
- Hold for 30 seconds.
- Next, let the underside of the toes spread and come up onto the ball of the foot as far as your foot will allow.
- Hold for 30 seconds.
- Repeat on the opposite foot.

Sit or stand in a place where it is easy to balanace

....

You decide how much weight to put down onto your feet during these exercises

....

Practice before you put your shoes on and after you take them off

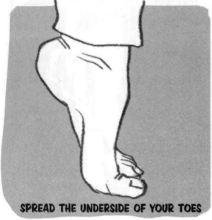

SPREAD THE UNDERSIDE OF YOUR TOES

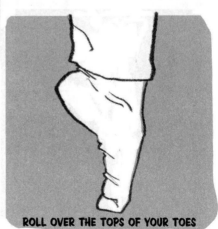

ROLL OVER THE TOPS OF YOUR TOES

NEVER LOSE HOPE

Thank you for picking up this book. I hope I've stirred something inside you to inspire you to get up and move more. Living a healthy life as a truck driver doesn't have to mean complicated programs. You can start with simple moves in the driver's seat, sleeper, and right outside your truck. And you can start today.

The only roadblock in your way to getting moving today is you thinking you can't. You now have a toolbox to add more movement and fitness into your day, throughout your day, every day. And before I go, I want to remind you that you can. You can do this. I believe in you. I hope you believe in yourself.

Take care of the body you live in because the replacement parts are never as good as the originals. Just remember: The next time you feel nervous or worried if someone will see you moving or exercising, you could be the reason they start taking better care of themselves, too, all because they saw you doing it first.

Now is the time to get up and move—
you are in the driver's seat.

Now is the time to get up and move—
you have all the tools you need.

Now is the time to get up and move—
your body is waiting for you to take action.

Now is the time to get up and move.

RESOURCES

This book is a simple way to get moving again as a truck driver. If you'd like to learn more about the foundations of this book, I recommend the following:

The Gray Institute Functional Applied Science, https://grayinstitute.com/

Gil Hidley "The Fuzz Speech" video, https://youtu.be/_FtSP-tkSug

Katy Bowman, *Move Your DNA: Restore Your Health through Natural Movement*

To purchase Mother Trucker Yoga's fitness strap or mini ball featured in this book, visit www.mothertruckeryoga.com/shop

For video instruction and printable PDF exercise guides, join the Mother Trucker Yoga LIFESTYLE JUMPSTART APP & Membership Platform at www.mothertruckeryoga.com

For detailed images of the squat, reach, bend, and rotation exercises mapped out in this book, visit www.mothertruckeryoga.com/truckingyogaexercises

We only recommend the best products to our customers, ones that we use ourselves. The following products have affiliate links and we may be paid a commission for sharing about their products:

BackShield, www.BackShield.com (use code MTY10 for 10% off)

Squatty Potty, https://amzn.to/36gQ1SR

ACKNOWLEDGMENTS

To my husband, Brian: Thank you for believing in me even before I fully believed in myself. Your unwavering support emotionally, physically, and financially has been one of the biggest reasons I am where I am today. I have spent more than half my life with you, and each year it just keeps getting better and better. You are the yin to my yang. And without you none of this would be possible.

Swami My Devananda: You were my first real yoga teacher, and it was you who taught me about the spiritual and internal importance of yoga. It was you who planted the seed for me to transform yoga into an everyday life experience. And it was you who made me realize that yoga could be the tool in my toolbox to help me in recovery. Thank you.

All my yoga students: You were more than just students, you were teachers for me as much as I was to you. Thank you for being the mirror, the platform, the believers I needed to find my own way on and off the yoga mat.

Julie: For believing in my message and telling me that I had a book. Also, thank you for helping me grow as a writer and bringing clarity and professionalism to my dream of having a published book with a real publisher.

My trucking family: You know who you are. To the handful of you who took me in and believed in my message. Thank you from the bottom of my heart. I am forever grateful.

ABOUT THE AUTHOR

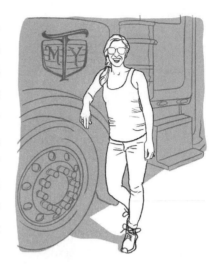

Hope Zvara is a yoga, movement, and lifestyle expert, speaker, and author. She has been in the yoga and fitness industry since 2003, helping others purposefully excel by focusing on three main areas: breath, body, and belief. She is known for her motivational personality and unique ability to break movements down and explain even the smallest of sensations and experiences.

In 2017 Hope stepped into the trucking industry ready to change the industry standard and show drivers how health, fitness, and trucking can go together. In 2019 she closed her yoga studio, determined to take Mother Trucker Yoga to the next level and to set a new fitness and wellness standard for truck drivers and trucking companies to follow.

Hope has been featured in publications such as *Mind Body Green, Elephant Journal, Reader's Digest, Thrive Global, Total Shape, California Herald, Truckers News, 10-4 Magazine,* and *Freight Waves.* Hope was featured on the two-time Emmy-nominated show STARTUP (2021), where she shared her entrepreneurial journey and how Mother Trucker Yoga is making an impact in the trucking industry. *Disrupt Magazine* also named her one of the "Top 30 Female Entrepreneurs to Look Out For in 2022." She has spoken on dozens of physical and online stages, podcasts, and radio shows across the country.

In 2020 Hope took to the open road to introduce her trucker-focused pain relief cream STIFF Mother Trucker, which quickly took a place in the pain relief market. Her highly acclaimed product is made with twelve all-natural ingredients, is gluten-free, sulfate-free, artificial dye–free, paraben-free and 100 percent vegan. She believes STIFF Mother Trucker is a pain relief cream everyone can get behind by "telling your toughest pains to hit the road." And STIFF Mother Trucker is proudly made in the USA. Hope's pain formula is catching the attention of many, as it was featured in Tori Spelling's (from *Beverly Hills 90210*) Celebrity Gift Box and listed in the *Forbes* "Holiday Gift Guide 2020: The Best Gifts for a Luxury Road Trip." It can be found at Love's Travel Shops across the country.

CONTACT HOPE

Visit Mother Trucker Yoga's online membership site for drivers and companies, sign up for her newsletter, and learn about her new Lifestyle JUMPSTART APP:
www.MotherTruckerYoga.com

To order books for your trucking school, company or event:
www.MotherTruckerYoga.com/contact

Explore Mother Trucker Yoga's 20-minute workout videos, audio meditation downloads, and fitness products:
www.MotherTruckerYoga.com/shop

Book Hope for your next conference or company wellness programming and seminars (virtual and in-person):
www.MotherTruckerYoga.com/contact

To learn more about or purchase STIFF Mother Trucker pain relief cream, visit www.STIFFMotherTrucker.com

Find Hope and Mother Trucker Yoga on social media:
LinkedIn: www.linkedin.com/in/hope-zvara-77572935
Instagram: @mothertruckeryoga
Facebook: @mothertruckeryoga
YouTube: www.youtube.com/mothertruckeryoga

Websites:
www.MotherTruckerYoga.com
www.STIFFMotherTrucker.com
www.HopeZvara.com